# SUPER ROOTS

A tribute to the Asian grandmother I never had.

Photography by Patricia Niven

# SUPER ROOTS

## Cooking with healing spices to boost your mood

Tanita de Ruijt

*Hardie Grant*

BOOKS

# CONTENTS

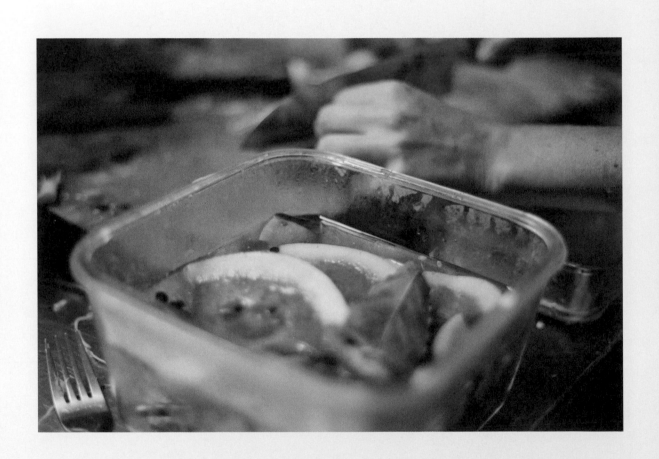

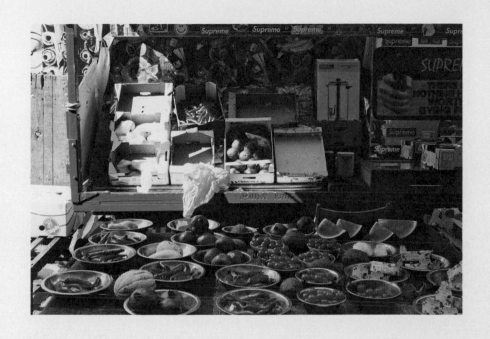

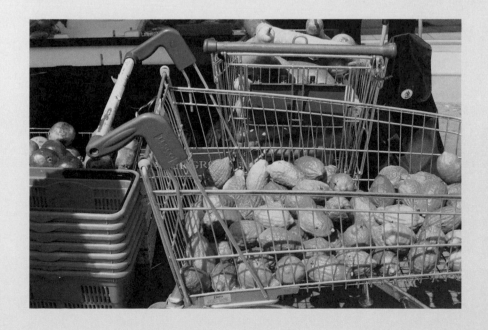

# A DELICIOUSLY DIFFERENT VIEW OF FOOD & WELLNESS

# ONE THAT'S BEEN ESTABLISHED FOR THOUSANDS OF YEARS

# INTRODUCTION

I've been inspired by Indonesia's culture – its traditional medicinal knowledge, culinary wisdom and beauty secrets – for years. The Indonesians rely on local ingredients such as herbs, barks, roots and spices to maintain a general sense of wellbeing and to enhance their beauty.

Eating and learning to cook their local food is what made me realise just how humble these ingredients were, and how easy it would be to incorporate more of them into my diet in a satisfying, synergistic and sustainable way. It also made me look and feel absolutely brilliant.

It's not only Indonesia that has inspired me; I have learned (and continue to learn) tremendous amounts about living well from various ancient food cultures all over Asia.

Koreans, for example, believe that good health and ailments arise from the quality of the food we eat and the way that we eat it. Traditional Korean recipes capture many of the wellness 'trends' we see today, including fermentation and the use of unprocessed ingredients.

The ability to boost one's 'wellbeing' is also one of the most popular marketing claims for food products in South Korea, even today. Home remedies and recipes for colds, hangovers and low energy have been used for hundreds, if not thousands, of years.

From alkalising and gut-soothing kimchi pickles and miso soup to anti-inflammatory ginger- and turmeric-infused everything, our eating habits are already influenced by so many Eastern traditions. We are only beginning to catch up with what these cultures have been practising for centuries

Discovering these traditions and reinvigorating them is what makes me tick. You'll often find me roaming the supermarket aisles of Chinatown – one of my favourite pastimes – or slurping a comforting pho noodle soup at a humble Vietnamese canteen. You won't find me at trendy juice bars.

With this book, my aim is to preserve and help simplify the Eastern principles that have sustained healthy people for centuries. I want to help you incorporate more functional ingredients into your diet, effortlessly and deliciously, through chapters filled with recipes and ideas to suit your mood.

## Renewing culture, restoring health

Traditional food knowledge refers to a cultural practice of sharing food, recipes and cooking skills and techniques and passing down that collective wisdom through generations.

When we think of healthy diets and people, the Japanese immediately spring to mind. Research tells us that the Japanese, particularly the people of Okinawa, have the healthiest diet and are the longest living people in the world.

Okinawa is the Hawaii of Japan — an exotic, easy-going group of islands with balmy weather, palm trees and white sandy beaches. This Pacific archipelago known as Ryukyu has maintained its reputation for nurturing extreme longevity for almost a thousand years.

Geographically, the Ryukyu Islands lie directly between Japan and China, and their traditional cuisine only started to develop during the trade era of the 14th century when the Chinese emperor of the new Ming Dynasty sent multiple Chinese diplomats to settle there. The Okinawans saw this as a tremendous opportunity to learn from the greatest superpower in the region – China.

The Okinawan diet was hugely influenced by China's ancient ideas of longevity achieved through diet. Okinawans use the term *nuchi gusui* to define their traditional cuisine, '*nuchi*' representing life, '*gusui*', medicine. In Chinese culture, there is no clear distinction between food and medicine.

The people of Okinawa also rely on herbs and spices to support their general wellbeing. They use them in two ways: first, as cures for specific ailments and as preventative medicine. They make their own herb and spice tinctures and tonics such as turmeric tea and mixtures of ingredients such as hibiscus flowers, mint and lemongrass; potions for treating minor ailments such as colds – a practice I explore in my first book, *Tonic*. The second way they use them is connected to the maintenance of good health and the enhancing of culinary flavours, for everyday consumption in the dishes they prepare – the topic of this book.

China's traditional and medicinal food knowledge also had a profound influence on its neighbouring countries such as Korea, Japan, Southeast Asia, India and Persia. It is an element of their healing system, known as Traditional Chinese Medicine (TCM), which developed around 3,000 years ago. This system was considered the world's most advanced system of medicine until the European renaissance.

Neighbouring traditional systems, such as Indonesian Jamu and Indian Ayurveda, have many similarities to TCM's core principles, yet they have evolved to suit the culture and native agriculture of their local environments.

These core principles are therefore also applicable beyond Asia. We too can incorporate these ideas and rituals into our own diets, using the functional foods that grow locally here in the West, as well as those we have available to us from the East thanks to globalisation and the modern spice trade.

In the West, we base the healthiness of our meals on the scientific quantities of proteins, fats, calories, carbohydrates, vitamins, antioxidants and other nutritional properties they contain. We do not, however, consider the quality of that food source, or take a person's unique constitution, mood or environment (season) into account.

The Eastern approach, on the other hand, is not one-size-fits-all but, instead, considers each person distinctly, viewing them as a whole: body, mind and spirit. The focus of Chinese medicine is also the quality and flavour of the food as opposed to its quantity.

By eating the correct foods for your constitution and environment, you're feeding your body what it craves and needs to be healthy and balanced. This will vary from one person to the other and it requires a level of intuition that is attained by practising several key principles and rituals.

### A key ingredient: mothers

There is a lot of reliable wisdom in culture – it's been teaching us how to eat for millennia. Culture represents thousands of years of trial and error and accumulated wisdom. It is a tool for wellness that we currently don't value enough.

Culture is also just another word for our mothers. We turn to our mothers for guidance. Our mothers tell us what to eat, how to eat and how much to eat. It's the wisdom of our family tribe. It's unique to every single individual and family, yet united by our community and environment.

Humble, comforting meals that are cooked at home using natural ingredients, usually by our mothers, are a representation of our mother's love. Nothing beats it; it is a personal definition of home, health, comfort, trust and nostalgia.

Cooking real food at home is the beginning of health and happiness. When you cook, you won't just want to cook for yourself, but for other people too. Sharing meals with others at the table is the beginning of a necessary cultural revolution in which we can take on the important role of the cultural 'mother' and continue to pass on vital wisdoms

### Quality

Home-cooked meals also guarantee one very important thing: quality.

We spend a lot of time questioning whether a food is healthy or not, sometimes even alienating entire food groups. Yet, according to traditional Chinese medicine, every food is nutritious, and as long as a healthy person doesn't eat too much of any one food, nothing can be unhealthy. The healthiness of an ingredient is determined by quality and processing, not its quantity.

Good-quality, unprocessed foods are super – they offer all of the nutrients and flavours we could possibly ever need. Nutrients and flavours keep us healthy and satisfied, which naturally also reduce the quantity of food we eat. Once we start to appreciate the beauty of well-grown, good-quality produce and the tastefulness of it, it's hard to look back. Processed foods become tasteless and no longer keep us full or satisfied.

Cooking traditional recipes from various food cultures of the East has helped me understand how to prepare and eat these quality ingredients correctly. With every traditional recipe I encounter, I learn more about powerful synergistic combinations and preserving methods that have sustained healthy people for centuries; how to get the most out of every bite in the most resourceful and delicious ways possible.

### Healing tastes

The secret to the deliciousness of all Asian food is the balancing act between flavours. Thai food is a brilliant example of a cuisine that understands this balance. Each dish, or shared meal as a whole, is made up of all five tastes – a perfect harmony between sweetness, sourness, saltiness, spiciness, and bitterness that leave us feeling wonderfully satisfied and reinvigorated (pages 29–37).

While there's no doubt that a perfect balance of tastes is essential in achieving ultimate deliciousness, did you know that flavour also happens to be deliciously healing?

**Flavour plays a fundamental role in all ancient Eastern systems of medicine. The taste of an ingredient doesn't just exist for our pleasure: it also has particular functions inside the body. Each taste represents one of the five elements, and one of our vital organs. The taste of an ingredient has tonic-like and remedial qualities that support specific organs. Flavour can stimulate our digestive system, help flush out common colds, calm inflammation, energise and detoxify the body.**

Incorporating more restorative flavours from good-quality ingredients into my meals every day makes me feel content and satisfied: balanced between body and mind. Happy.

This system of flavours is a tool to meet the ultimate goal of Chinese medicine: bringing the body into balance. Along with things like meditation and exercise, food and flavour are one of the most accessible and intuitive ways to find and keep this balance.

Sweetness is actually considered the most central and important flavour when it comes to nourishing the body, and should always make up the foundation of our meal. We forget that carbohydrates such as grains, vegetables, pulses (legumes) and seeds are all sweet, which actually makes the balancing act quite simple. Layering small amounts of salty, spicy, sour and bitter foods on top of that foundation creates a perfectly balanced plate.

What's more, focussing on flavour not only creates balance, it also brings us in harmony with the seasons. Seasonal ingredients happen to have the perfect flavours to help us through that particular time of year – nature truly is fascinating in this sense.

Lastly, combining flavours creates synergistic effects on the bioactivity of these foods, which is vital when it comes to absorbing their benefits. Flavours that grow together, as well as taste good together, naturally help to increase each other's bio-availability (i.e. ginger, turmeric and black pepper and coconut oil, or even tomatoes and olive oil). It's yet another reason why I'm fascinated with time-tested, traditional recipes that taste delicious and are proving to be incredibly healing, too.

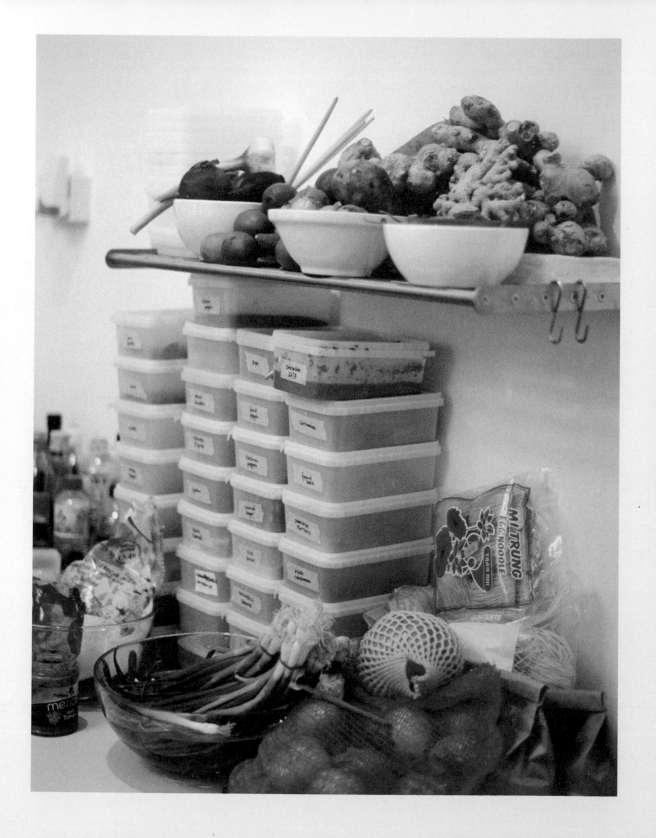

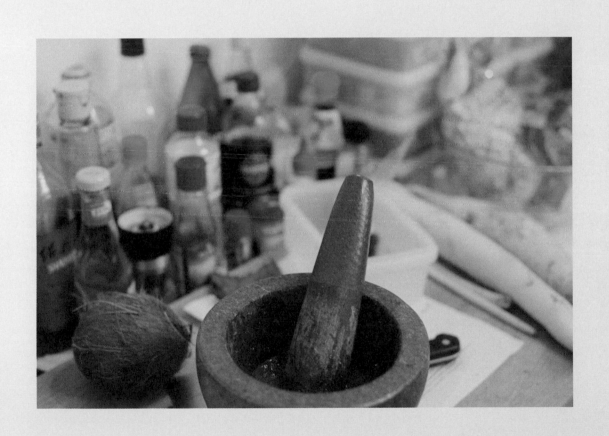

# COOK'S NOTES

*Before you begin, here are some scribbles, tips and pointers on some of the more unusual utensils, processes and ingredients used in this book. Most ingredients can be found in Chinese or general Asian supermarkets if not in your local supermarket.*

## EQUIPMENT

**Pestle and mortar** – This tool comes in all shapes and sizes. I prefer to pound my ingredients using a pestle and mortar, as it's much easier than chopping, and creates great tastes and textures. When a recipe calls for a spice paste or minced garlic or ginger for example, assume I've bashed it up into a paste in my mortar. When using a pestle and mortar, start by pounding the hardest ingredients first. Always add a pinch of salt to help break down the ingredients as you pound.

Alternatively, chopping these ingredients up really finely will also work. You can use the flat part of the blade of your knife to mush them up after chopping them really small. You can also use a blender if you're short for time.

**Julienne peeler** – In my opinion, the Kiwi brand makes the best julienne peeler. These save a lot of time and effort, and create lovely looking strips of vegetables. You can buy them online.

**Cleavers and chef knives** – Essential. Invest in one or two good-quality knives. They are perfect for chopping, mashing and peeling ingredients with.

**Woks** – Not essential, but wonderful to cook all sorts of dishes in, depending on the size. The wok is probably the most versatile pan I own! Woks are originally Chinese, but are used predominantly for frying in Bali.

**Blenders** – Nutribullets are great for blending spice pastes and sambals with.

## TECHNIQUES & TASTING

All the recipes in this book are designed to balance sweet, salty, sour, spicy and bitterness. It's important to include all of these elements into every dish or meal, but it's also important to adapt dishes to your personal taste. Make a dish spicier if that's what you fancy – it's your meal after all.

## PICKLING & FERMENTING

All things fermented and somewhat funky require wild yeasts that co-exist with plenty of other microorganisms, including a substantial amount of acetic acid bacteria. These are essential for developing refreshing pickles, but there can be other less welcome bacteria that can develop in a batch too. If your pickle or ferment smells bad, or starts to grow mould, get rid of it and start again.

## STERILISATION

Sterilise any jars or containers you plan to make pickles or ferments in. It prevents any nasty bacteria from interfering with them.

To sterilise your jars or containers, clean them in a white vinegar solution. Fill a large bowl with a solution of half hot water and half white vinegar. Let them soak in this solution for 20 minutes. While they are soaking, give them a good scrub with a brush. Dry them thoroughly.

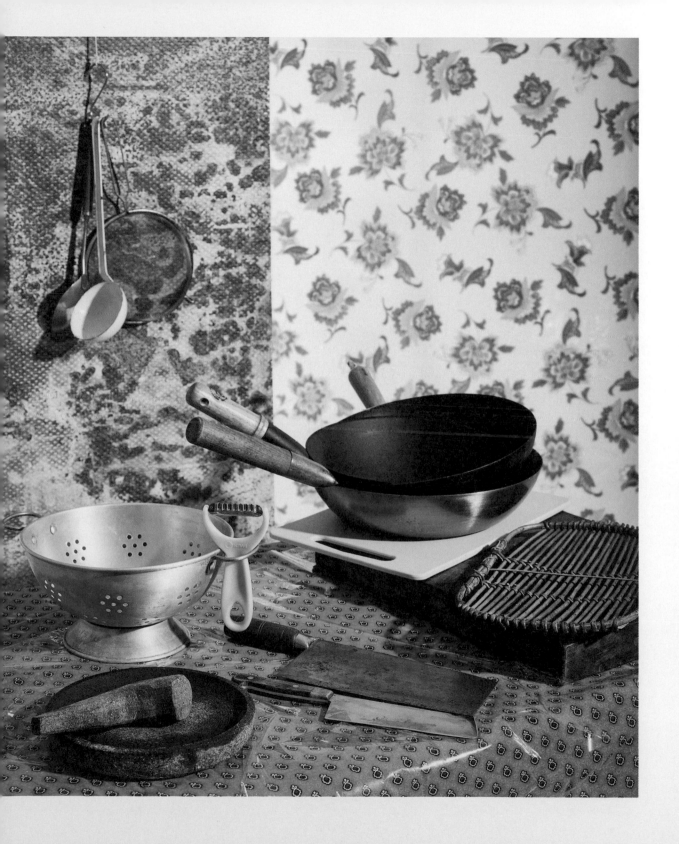

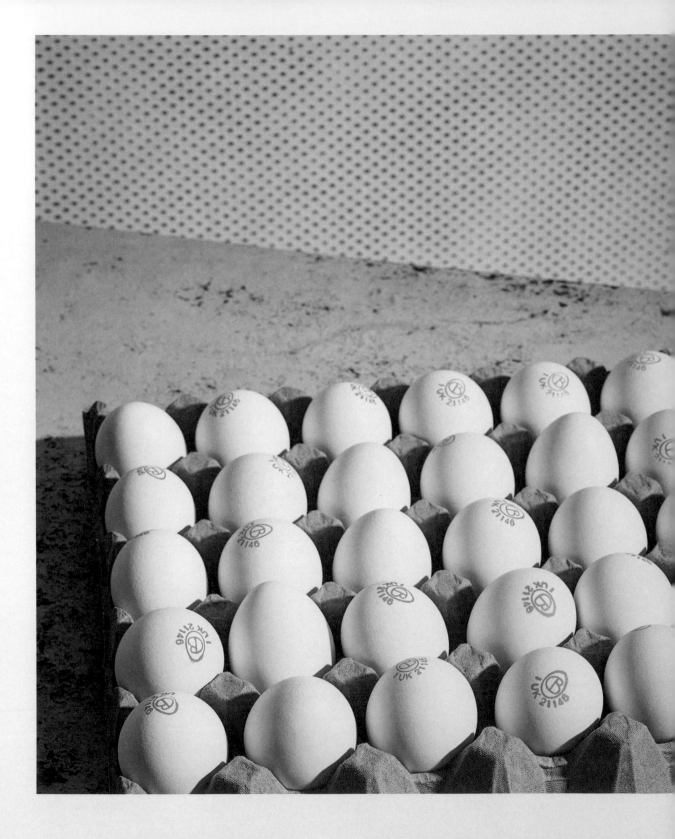

# INGREDIENTS

**Anchovies** – I use these in a lot of my recipes, to replicate the flavour of shrimp paste, belacan or to add a dash of umami to my dish. Anchovies are much easier to find than belacan. If you'd rather not use anchovies, try a splash of fish sauce, soy sauce or a pinch of salt instead.

**Black rice vinegar** – This malty, woody and smoky rice vinegar from China is made with black rice. If you can't find it, you can substitute it with equal parts apple cider vinegar and balsamic vinegar.

**Chilli** – There's a lot of confusion around chillies, as they are available in so many different forms. In this book, I tell you exactly what kind you need. Please do try to look for those exact fresh or dry chillies I refer to, as using alternatives will have a significant impact on your dish. All fresh chillies should be washed, wiped dry and have green stalks removed.

**Coconut milk** – Always use full-fat (whole) coconut milk. 'Light' or 'low fat' coconut milk is no good: it has been diluted with water, so you're getting less coconut goodness. If you want a lighter milk, just add more water to it. I never shake a tin of coconut milk. Open your tin of coconut milk and scoop out all (or some) of the solidified coconut part first. Let this dissolve into your dish, then add the water in the tin afterwards. This gives you maximum control of the dish's consistency.

**Coconut oil** – Use cheap coconut oil for frying or cooking. I keep 'virgin' coconut oil in the bathroom for my skin.

**Coconut sugar** – This is my favourite type of sugar to cook with. I buy mine in cylindrical blocks, but ground coconut sugar is good too. If you can't find it, use any unrefined sugar you like.

**Ginger** – Always peel fresh ginger.

**Kecap manis** – This is sweetened soy sauce from Indonesia, and it's a staple condiment in my kitchen. Buy it at your local Asian supermarket or online. ABC Sweet Soy Sauce (Kecap Manis) is what you're looking for.

**Miso paste** – I usually use white miso paste in my recipes as the flavour is more mild. Feel free to experiment with others, but be mindful to balance the saltiness – the darker the paste, the saltier it is.

**Olive oil** – Use bland, olive oil for frying and infusing Asian spices. Save extra-virgin olive oil to enjoy for its taste!

**Perfect eggs** – Steaming eggs for 7 minutes makes for a perfectly cooked egg. Find a pan that will fit the amount of eggs you want to cook in one layer on the bottom. Fill it with about 1 cm (½ in) of water, place on the hob over high heat, wait for it to start boiling, then turn down the heat to low. Pop a lid on the pan, and start your timer for 7 minutes.

**Rice** – You can use any kind of rice to make the recipes in this book. Black, red, white, brown – they are all good, as long as you eat a variety. White rice has already been milled, so doesn't need to cook for as long as black, red and brown varieties, which need to be soaked in water in order for the outer bran to be broken down. *Always wash your rice before cooking.* Here are my preferred varieties:

**> Black, brown, red rice** – Overnight method: Soak the rice overnight. Combine 1 part rice with 1.5 parts water. Start with the rice in cold water, let it come to the boil, then place a lid on the pan and reduce the heat to low. Let the rice cook until the water has been completely absorbed.

Quick, 30-minute soak method: Soak for 30 minutes. Then 1 part rice to 2 parts water. Start with cold water, let this come to a boil, place a lid on your pan and reduce heat to low. Let this cook until the water has fully absorbed.

**> Long-grain white rice (i.e. jasmine, basmati)** – 1 part rice to 1 part water. Start with the rice in cold water, let it come to the boil, then place a lid on the pan and reduce the heat to low. Let the rice cook until the water has been completely absorbed.

**> Short-grain white rice** – 1 part rice to 1 part water. Start with the rice in cold water, let it come to the boil, then place a lid on the pan and reduce the heat to low. Let the rice cook until the water has been completely absorbed.

**Roasted sesame paste** – The most common sesame paste we find is Middle Eastern tahini, the unroasted kind that is used to make hummus. In China, sesame paste is roasted, so it's crucial to recognise the difference to create authentic flavour. Light sesame paste is usually unroasted. Dark sesame paste is roasted. These are both available in health food stores or online if you can't find them in your local supermarket. Or, you can make your own by simply dry-grinding sesame seeds in a pestle and mortar.

**Salt** – Use unrefined salts, like sea salts, Himalayan pink salts or black salts (*kala namak*) which are salty and have a sulphurous eggy taste and smell to them, and are pink in colour (see photo opposite). Perfect for substituting eggs if you're vegan and an easy way to add the depth and flavour of eggs to dishes without having to use them. Salts are also packed with minerals.

**Soy sauce** – Soy sauce is unfortunately not gluten-free, but if you want to make a dish gluten-free you can substitute with tamari or coconut aminos.

**Tamarind** – Blocks or slabs of tamarind have been slightly fermented and therefore keep for a long time. Look for unsalted tamarind blocks that are quite soft, pliable and squidgy. Before you start cooking, dissolve as much tamarind as the recipe requires in warm water, then strain that dissolved tamarind water through a fine-mesh sieve before using. You can buy tamarind blocks in Asian supermarkets or as a concentrate in regular supermarkets. If using tamarind concentrate (look for ones not packed with preservatives), there's no need to dilute it further with water. Add it to your dish to taste, as it will always be somewhat sourer than tamarind water.

**Tempeh** – Tempeh is a fermented soy bean cake from Indonesia, which makes a super-delicious vegetarian source of protein. It is available in most health food stores and Asian supermarkets. Those produced in Holland (if buying in the UK) are usually the most fresh and authentic.

**Turmeric** – For the best flavour and medicinal qualities, use fresh turmeric. You can store fresh turmeric root in the freezer, and pull a piece out when you need it. It only needs to thaw for a minute or two before it's ready to slice or grate it straight from frozen. There's no need to peel turmeric, just wash it properly.

*2 cm (¾ in) fresh turmeric = 1 tbsp freshly grated turmeric = 1 tsp ground turmeric.*

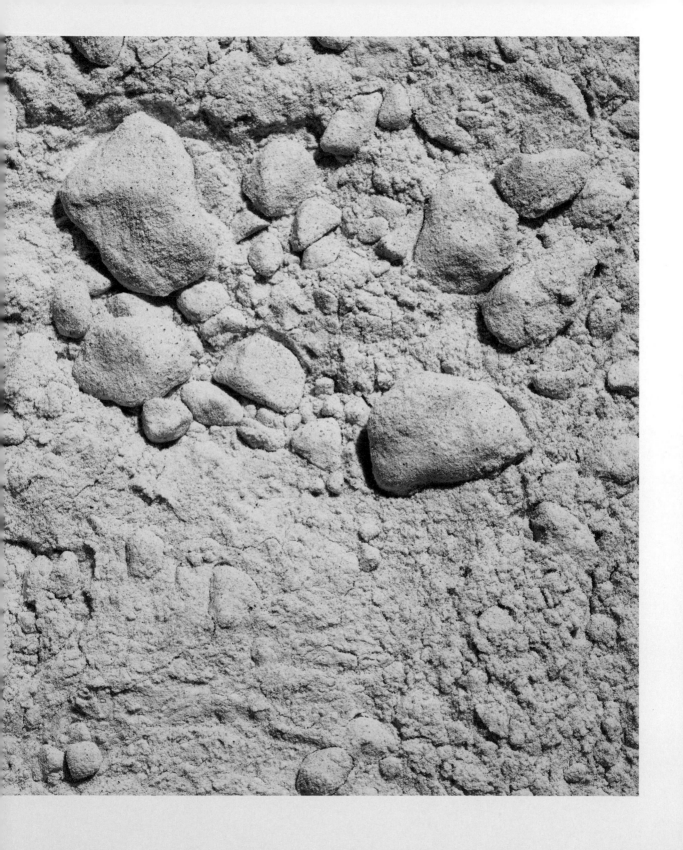

# TOP 12 HEALING TASTE- MAKERS

*A collection of handy kitchen cupboard staples to use to your medicinal advantage.*

## 1. BLACK PEPPER

According to Ayurveda, the pungency and heat of black pepper work to help metabolise food as it is digested in our system. Its warming qualities also help to clear congestion in the respiratory system. Use for indigestion, sinus congestion, excess toxin build-up, fever, sluggish metabolism and obesity.

## 2. CARDAMOM

Known as 'the queen of spices', cardamom is related to ginger. Like ginger, it's good for improving digestion, soothing stomach pains and relieving gas. Its warming properties also help to cleanse the body, and improve circulation. You will have to break open the pods to discover its plethora of health benefits.

## 3. CHILLI: FRESH OR DRIED

The heat you feel from cayenne pepper and chilli powder comes from capsaicin, a compound that has been shown to invigorate the blood, clear the nasal passages and thin mucus. Fresh chillies also pack more vitamin C than oranges.

## 4. CINNAMON

An antibacterial spice found in most households, cinnamon increases general vitality, warms the body, counteracts congestion, improves digestion, relieves menstrual cramping and improves circulation. Look for Sri Lankan 'Ceylon cinnamon' (*Cinnamomum verum*), also known as 'true cinnamon', not cassia bark (Chinese cinnamon, *Cinnamomum cassia*). Grate the bark straight into your concoctions.

## 5. CLOVE

Cloves are the aromatic flower buds of a medicinal tree once indigenous to the Indonesian 'spice islands'. Also found in the spice racks of most homes, cloves are known to have antiseptic, anaesthetic, anti-inflammatory, warming, soothing and flatulence-relieving properties.

## 6. CUMIN

The cumin seed was once thought to promote love and fidelity – it was thrown around at weddings, and soldiers were even sent off to battle with a fresh loaf of cumin-seed bread. It's traditionally used as a carminative, to help settle the stomach, and ease bloating and trapped wind.

## 7. GARLIC

Aphrodisiac, currency, food, medicine, vampire repellent – garlic has had several uses in many cultures for thousands of years. Its pungent sulphurs and antibacterial and anti-inflammatory properties are used to prevent colds and flu and treat a wide range of conditions and diseases.

## 8. GINGER

The best-known member of the family: primarily for its flavour, but also for protecting and promoting a healthy digestive system. It's one of the most ancient medicinal plants used in Chinese, Ayurvedic and Indonesian medicine. In Asia, ginger is known to warm the body, ease nausea, rev up the appetite and digestion, help ward off any aches and pains, as well as restore strength to those suffering from illness. Steeped hot ginger teas help relieve symptoms of cold and flu. When combined with turmeric, its effects multiply. The skin can be left on, as long as it is rinsed thoroughly.

## 9. LEMONGRASS

An aromatic healer with a distinct lemony flavour and citrussy aroma, lemongrass is nature's paracetamol: it reduces pain and inflammation; helps to bring down high fevers; and relieves headaches. It's known as 'fevergrass' in Jamaica. Lemongrass also helps to restore our vital systems, including digestion, respiration, excretion and the nervous system. Heavily bruise the white part of this grass root to unlock its potential.

## 10. ONION

Onions have been used to reduce inflammation and heal infections for centuries. They're also one of the healthiest foods you can eat. A natural antihistamine, onions are also rich in vitamin C, sulphuric compounds, flavonoids and other phytochemicals that can soothe the throat and clear stuffed-up nasal passages. An onion a day may help keep the doctor away.

## 11. STAR ANISE

Used in traditional Chinese medicine to fight flu by clearing mucous from the respiratory tract, this spice is effective in fighting viral, bacterial or fungal infections, as well as inflammation. It's also a common ingredient in medicinal teas, to treat coughs and chest infections. The seeds can be chewed before meals to stimulate the appetite, or afterwards to relieve gas and bloating.

## 12. TURMERIC

Turmeric is king when it comes to spice. Its yellow colour has long been considered sacred in the Eastern world. Yellow symbolises the sun – a source of light, energy and growth – which is why this colour is associated with royalty and is believed to offer protection from evil spirits throughout Asia.

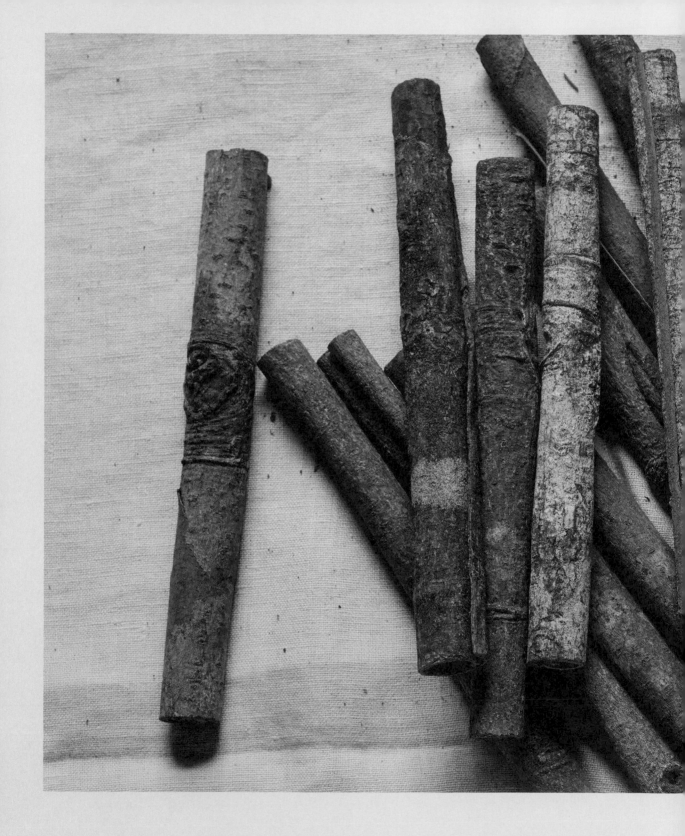

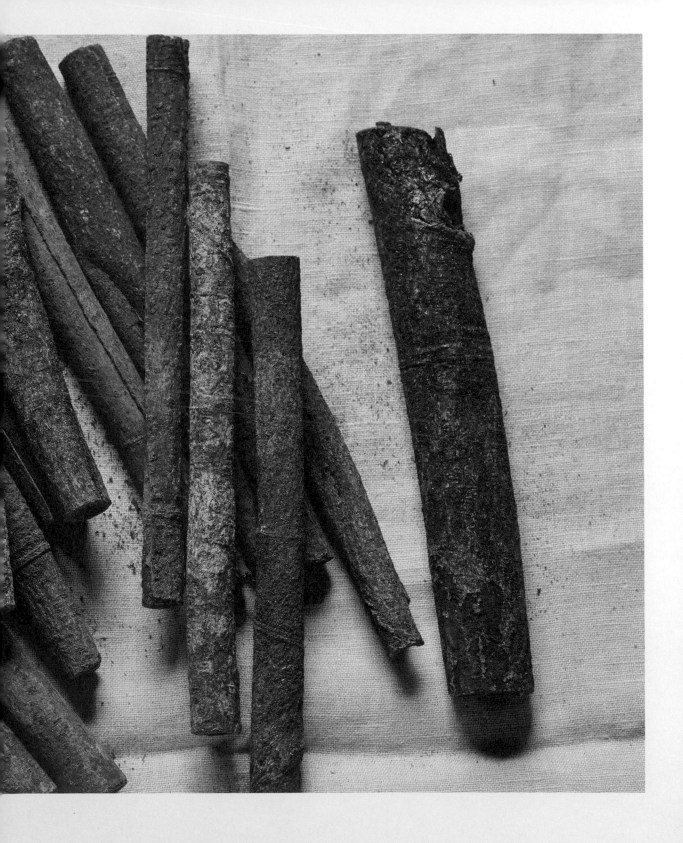

# RECIPES TO SUIT YOUR MOOD

It's about simple observation: tuning in to how you feel and considering what recipes combinations will put you back on track, quickly. There is wisdom in your cravings, and also in traditional cuisine.

Although making everything from scratch is rewarding, it's not necessary in order to cook the recipes in this book. High-quality shop-bought ingredients – from good-quality beef stock to chilli oil – can be bought and used in place of the homemade ingredients in the pantry section (pages 42–73).

Due to inspirations from the East, all the recipes are naturally dairy-free, and predominantly gluten-free. Almost all of the recipes can also be adapted to become vegetarian, and some to become vegan, too.

The next few pages focus on the various characteristics of ingredients and how, with a bit of thought, you can create delicious meals to suit your mood and boost your health.

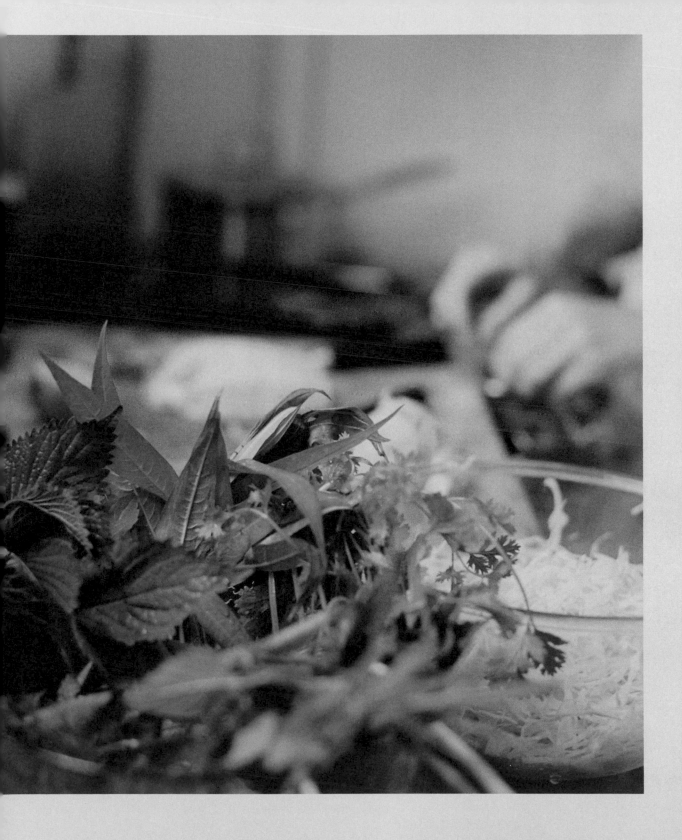

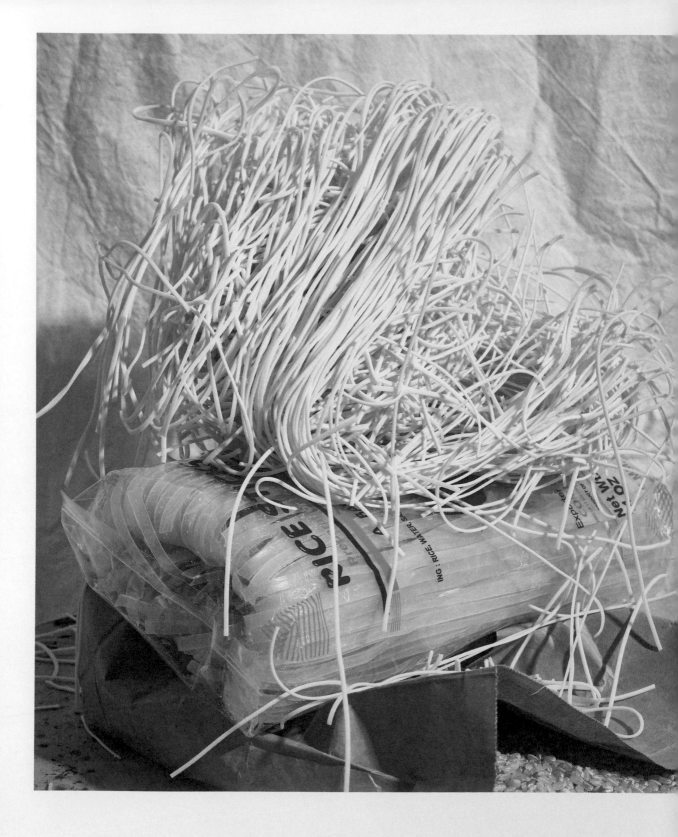

# SWEET
# & STARCHY

**Represents earth**

-

**Important in late summer**

-

**Warming/energising/strengthening**

-

**Fights cold and flu**

-

**Supports the spleen and stomach**

Sweet ingredients such as rice are used for healing in Chinese medicine. Sweetness constitutes carbohydrates such as grains, vegetables, pulses (legumes) and fruits. They are synonymous with tonifying and strengthening the body, they form part of our basic needs; our roots. Their flavour is both energising for the body and relaxing for the mind and nervous system. Sweet foods are also said to soothe heated emotions including anger and impatience, as well as calm nervous thoughts and anxieties that sit in our stomachs. Feeling nervous, frail or weak? Be sweeter to yourself.

*Rice, Potatoes, Sweet Potatoes, Noodles, Barley, Spelt, Peanuts, Cashews, Chickpeas (garbanzos), Pulses, Legumes, Coconut Blossom Nectar, Honey, etc.*

# SALTY & UMAMI

**Represents water**

-

**Important in winter**

-

**Cooling/energising/helps hangovers**

-

**Supports the kidneys and bladder**

Naturally salty foods from quality sources are essential. Salty tastes go to the kidneys first. They help regulate mineral and fluid balance, which also happens to be a major function of the kidneys. They also help to strengthen our digestive systems and detoxify the body. Salty flavours help create movement within our bodies, counteracting sluggishness and tiredness, especially in winter. They are perfect for symptoms such as lack of energy, lower back pain, tired legs and poor memory.

*Mushrooms, Miso, Pickles, Salts, Seaweeds, Soy Sauce, etc.*

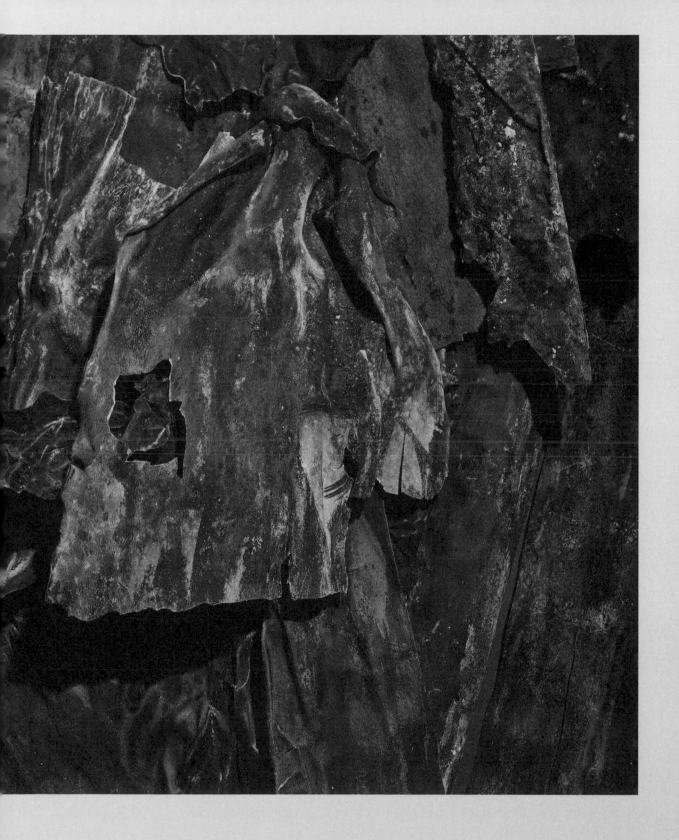

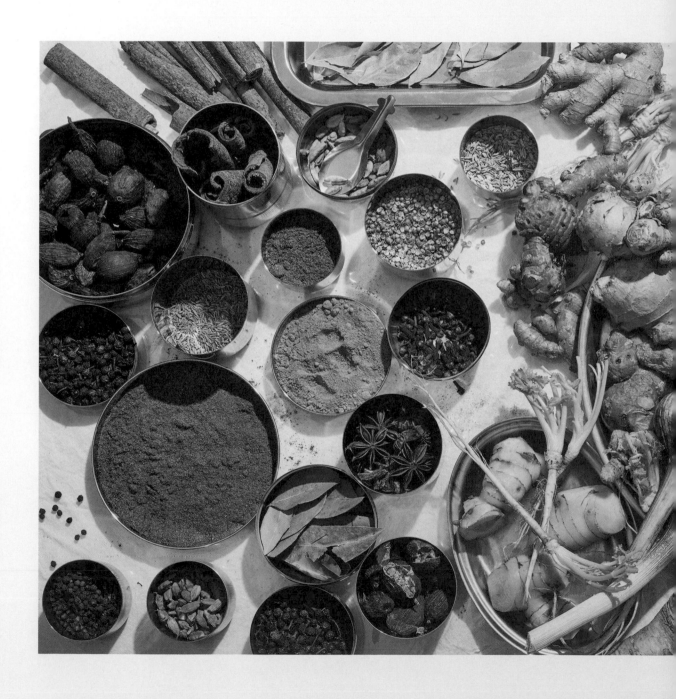

# PUNGENT & SPICY

Represents metal

-

Important in autumn

-

Warming/immunity boosting/source of prebiotics/prevents bloating/energising

-

Supports the lungs and large intestine

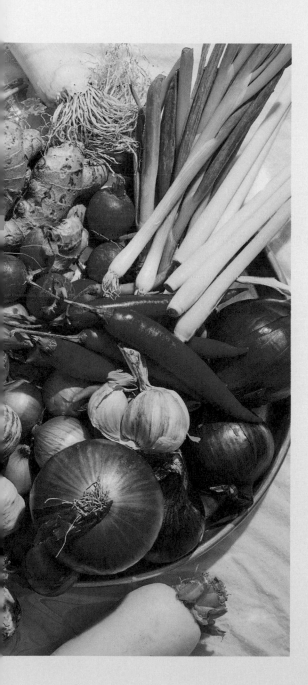

Traditional medicinal recipes usually constitute the trinity roots – garlic, onions and ginger. These roots are a powerful combination, good for just about anything that ails you. Pungent and spicy ingredients are powerful antioxidants, good blood purifiers, detoxifiers and immune-strengthening flavours.

Spicy ingredients are perfect for helping treat the symptoms of the common cold like sneezing, runny noses, coughs, headaches, body aches, feeling cold or a sore throat. Spicy tastes go straight to the lungs and can help to expel these symptoms from the body, especially in cold seasons. This is why Chinese medicine recommends adding some spicy flavours to your cooking in autumn to prep and boost your immune system to avoid colds and flu. See my Top 12 healing taste-makers on pages 22–23.

Our immune system also depends on a healthy gut. Raw alliums such as onions, as well as garlic, are also important sources of prebiotics – fibres that feed your gut bacteria – and are equally as important as probiotics from ferments and pickles.

Prebiotic fibre goes through the small intestine undigested and is fermented when it reaches the large colon. This fermentation process feeds the bacteria in our gut and helps to increase the number of good bacteria in our digestive systems.

Consider your gut to be a garden. You can add seeds – the probiotic bacteria from foods such as kimchi – yet the prebiotic fibre acts as the water and fertiliser that help the seeds grow and flourish.

*Bay Leaves, Black Cardamom, Black Pepper, Chillies, Cinnamon, Cloves, Coriander Seeds, Garlic, Onions, Ginger, Green Cardamom, Korean Chilli Powder, Lemongrass, Radishes, Szechuan Peppercorns, Turmeric, etc.*

# BITTER

**Represents fire**

-

**Important in summer**

-

**Cooling/calming/digestion/energising**

-

**Supports the heart and small intestine**

Eating bitter foods helps us stay cool on the inside and out. In Chinese medicine, bitter foods are recommended for people who suffer from heat-related symptoms: ulcers, mouth sores, anxiety and insomnia.

Bitter flavours also get our digestive juices flowing. They help to soothe gas, burping, bloating and indigestion. They also help to keep our appetites and sweet tooth in check, and prevent us from overindulging.

As a food lover with an interest in health, I'm always searching for the sweet spot; where delicious meets healthy. Herbs do that perfectly. Not only a source of bitterness, they add enticing aroma, flavour and colour to food, and have some pretty remarkable health benefits too. When you move past seeing these ingredients as simply a garnish, and start to recognise them for the culinary players that they are, a whole new world of healthy food opens up.

Herbs (as well as spices) have been used since ancient times for their medicinal properties. Their healthful value as an ingredient in food should not be underestimated: recent studies show that their benefits also apply when they are cooked and eaten as part of a meal (Chohan, 2014).

Lastly, herbs naturally help us cut back on salt, and are abundant with healthy polyphenols: a source of potent antioxidants and anti-inflammatory and anti-microbial effects.

*Basil, Chervil, Chives, Coriander Leaf (cilantro), Dill, Mint, Oregano, Parsley, Rocket (arugula), Rosemary, Sage, Tarragon, Thyme, etc.*

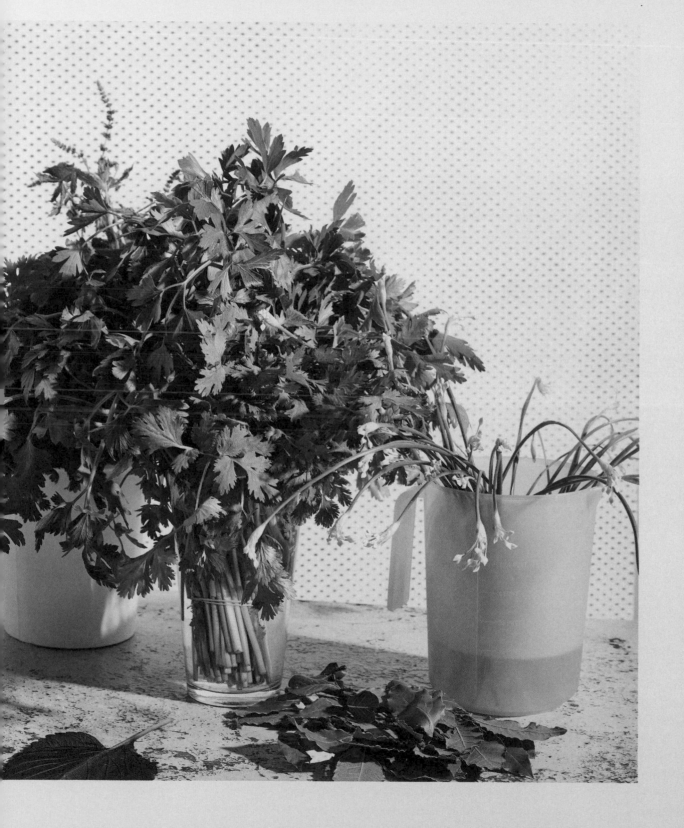

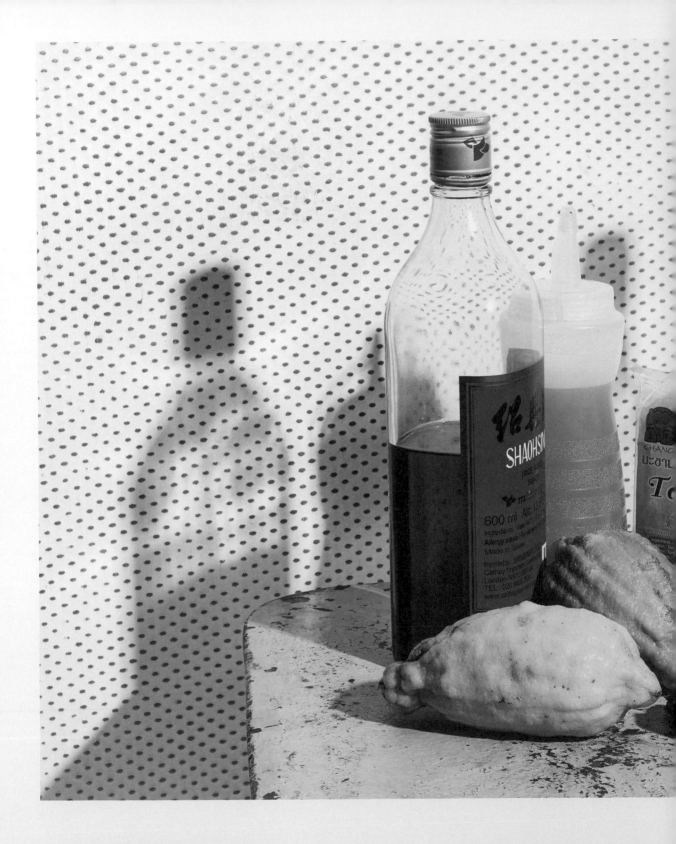

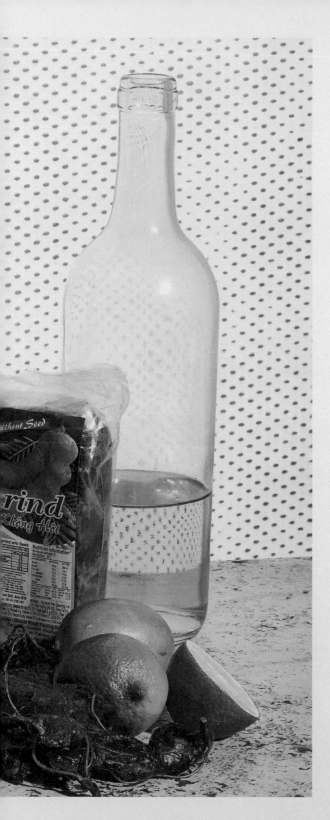

# SOUR

**Represents wood**

-

**Important in spring**

-

**Cooling/calming/supports digestion**

-

**Helps hangovers**

-

**Supports the liver and gallbladder**

Sour flavours support our liver. Their acidity helps trigger the digestive process, cutting through and breaking down fats and proteins from richer, greasy foods, and improving the absorption of essential nutrients.

Sourness also helps to calm the body. The liver is considered an important organ that dominates and determines our emotions. When the liver is muddled, the body will experience a lot of symptoms like being irritable and emotional. A drop of something sour will lend this overburdened organ a helpful jolt, while balancing your meal.

*Lemons, Limes, Pickles, Tamarind, Vinegars, etc.*

# BALANCE

*Chinese philosophers tell us to always take the 'golden means'; never take extremes. It's important not to eat too much, or too much of one thing (no matter how healthy it is), eat good-quality food and meals that are balanced in all flavours.*

The diagram opposite is of a basic meal in the everyday Korean diet, as recommended by the Korean government. It shows their idea of what constitutes a perfectly balanced plate. I use it as a guide to building my meals to make sure I have included most of the elements.

*Kuk* (boiled cooked rice and/or other grains, such as black rice, barley, sorghum, millets, and beans) is served alongside *bap* (a soupy broth), which helps in the swallowing and digestion of our food.

The meal is also accompanied by one type of *kimchi* (sour spicy pickle, page 52), one *namul* (seasoned leafy herbs), one vegetable dish (*banchan I*), and one high-protein dish (*banchan II*), usually made from fish or meat.

*Jang* (salty fermented sauces), such as Gochujang (page 63), are used to season food and stimulate one's appetite.

A variety of meals can be made using a variety of ingredients and cooking methods depending on the season, regions and one's preference and mood. The synergy of ingredients and methods allow for the flavours and nutrients to become well balanced and, above all, delicious.

## Food as therapy

Food really can heal in many ways: the actual process of cooking is calming and soothing, and allows for time and space to think and breathe. Sharing food with loved ones and even strangers makes one feel connected and encourages a sense of community. Then there's eating it too – my favourite part.

Cooking – as well as eating – doesn't just give me comfort and pleasure; it provides me with a sense of identity. The recipes in this book are an extension of me; my journey, the meals I've scoffed, the places I've been to; the things that make me feel well.

Although I am Dutch, I grew up on a Mediterranean diet in Spain, yet my identity was truly cultivated in Indonesia. Trips to the East, and the discovery of traditional systems of medicine such as Jamu, Ayurveda and traditional Chinese medicine have informed my relationship with food, and shaped my approach to eating well and cooking intuitively.

What I have learnt is that the recipe for wellbeing is considerably messy. There are unforeseen setbacks; it takes practise as well as intuition. Yet it is this simple act of exploration that revives my spirit and my interest in life. Sometimes food is what keeps me putting one foot in front of the other.

'Wellbeing' is a philosophy in motion. There is no quick fix, no shortcut; it's just a process. To me, the goal is the process. The more I practise cooking, the better cook I become, and in turn the better I eat and feel. To me, feeling well means finding your everyday *ikigai* – a reason for being. *Ikigai* is a concept from Japan, a prism for bringing satisfaction, happiness and meaning to one's life: it is usually found at the intersection of what you are good at and what you love doing. I found mine in the kitchen.

**A perfectly balanced plate**

1 - *Kuk (rice, which is sweet and starchy)*

2 - *Bap (soup/broth, which is usually salty)*

3 - *Namul (herbs/leaves, which are bitter)*

4 - *Banchan I (veggie dish, which is sweet and bitter)*

5 - *Banchan II (protein dish)*

6 - *Kimchi (something pickled or femented)*

7 - *Jang (fermented seasoning which is salty)*

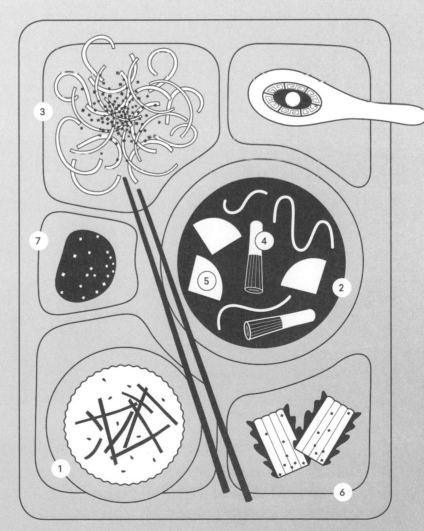

Make this entire meal on pg 106!

Reference: (Soon Hee Kim et al, 2016)

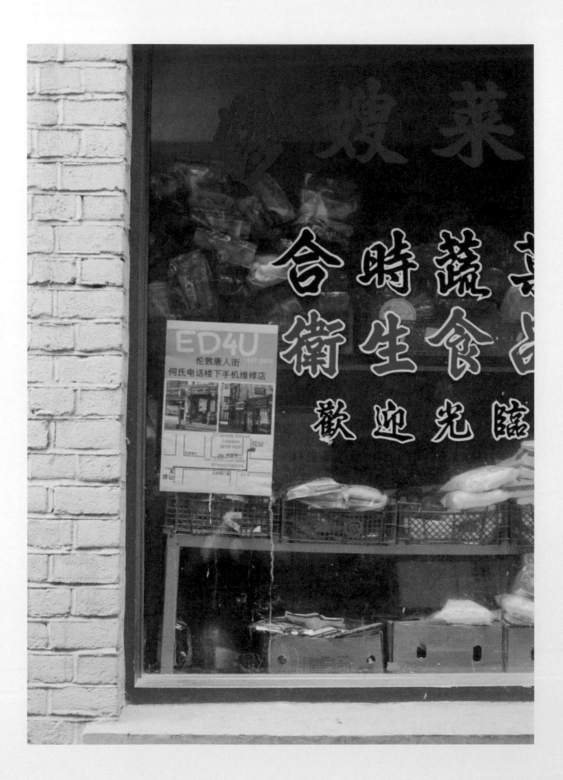

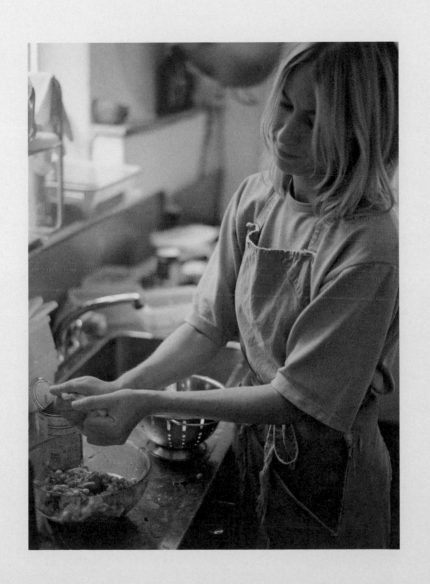

# PANTRY

CHOOSE YOUR FAVOURITE ELEMENTS
FROM THIS SECTION TO MAKE &
STOCK YOUR PANTRY. THIS WAY
YOU WILL ALWAYS HAVE THEM ON
HAND TO INSPIRE A NEW DISH OR
ADD EXTRA TONIC QUALITIES TO
YOUR OLD FAVOURITES.

# KOREAN TURMERIC PICKLE

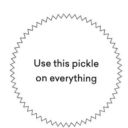

Use this pickle on everything

### Ingredients

400 g (14 oz) radishes (daikon is traditional), peeled and cut into thin slices

### Brine

300 ml (10 fl oz/1¼ cups) water

300 ml (10 fl oz/1¼ cups) apple cider vinegar or rice vinegar

90 g (3 oz/generous ⅓ cup) unrefined cane sugar

1 tbsp sea salt

2 garlic cloves, quartered

2 tsp ground turmeric

10 whole black peppercorns

2 bay leaves

*Turmeric pickle, or* **danmuji**, *is super easy to make and packed with tangy flavour, as well as nutritious ingredients, probiotics and anti-inflammatory goodness. This radish pickle is flavoured with garlic, turmeric, bay leaves and black pepper. I use apple cider vinegar instead of the traditional rice vinegar, but the choice is yours.*

### Method

Put all the ingredients for the brine in a large saucepan and mix this well. It should taste pungent and super sour. Bring it to the boil, then turn the heat off as soon as it starts to bubble. Add the sliced radishes and stir. Leave to cool.

Once cool, pack the pickle and the brine in a sterilised 1 litre (34 fl oz/4 cups) glass jar and keep it in the fridge for up to 4 months.

**Fills a 1 litre (34 fl oz/ 4 cup) jar**

**Vegetarian**

**Vegan**

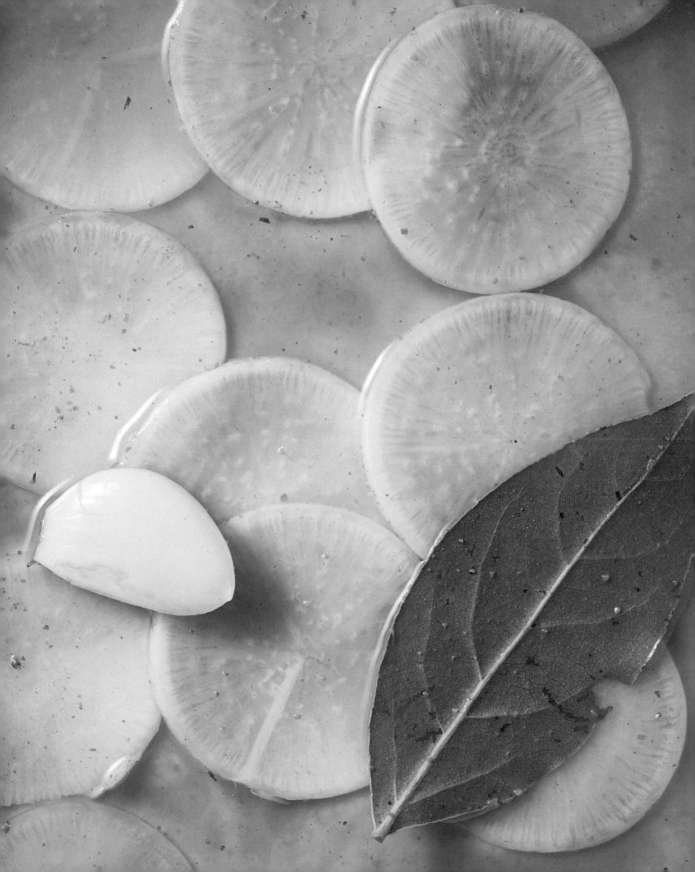

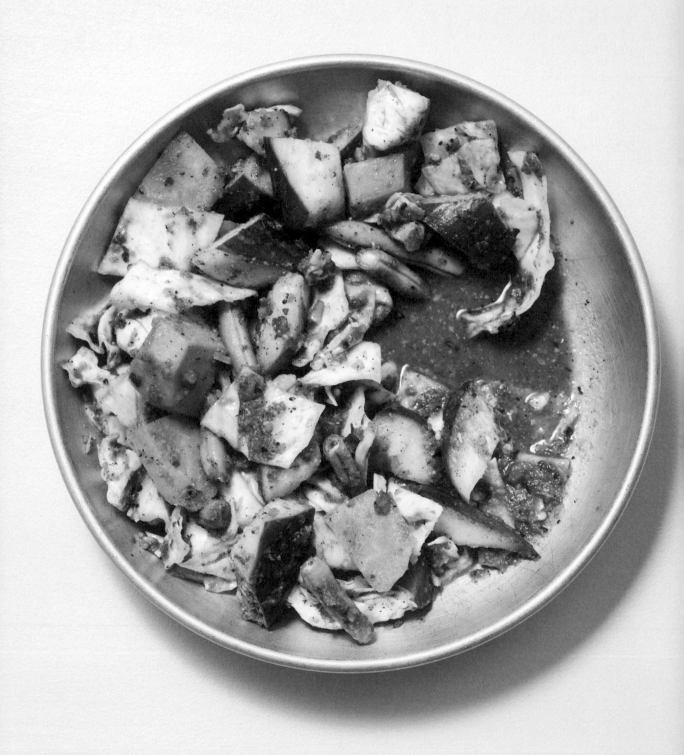

# TURMERIC PICKLE

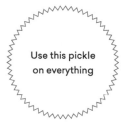

Use this pickle
on everything

*This colourful pickle – called **nyonya acar** – is from Penang, Malaysia, and uses fresh turmeric root. It's sweet, sour, crunchy, nutty, immunity-boosting – totally satisfying. And it's the easiest way to pile tonnes of vegetables onto any dish or into a sandwich when you're feeling a little lazy.*

Fills a 1 litre
(34 fl oz/
4 cup) jar

Vegetarian

Vegan

### Ingredients

1 tbsp sea salt

1 cucumber, peeled and cut into thick 3 cm- (1¼ in-) pieces, watery cores removed

⅓ pointed cabbage, roughly chopped

2 carrots, peeled and cut into thick 3 cm- (1¼ in-) pieces

handful of green beans, trimmed and cut into 3 cm- (1¼ in-) long pieces

2 tbsp toasted sesame seeds

2 tbsp roasted peanuts

3 tbsp coconut oil

50 ml (2 fl oz) rice vinegar or apple cider vinegar

50 ml (2 fl oz) water

1 tbsp unrefined sugar (I like to use coconut sugar)

### Spice Paste

5 small shallots

6 red bird's eye chillies

3 cm (1¼ in) piece of fresh turmeric

### Method

In a bowl, rub the salt into the prepped cucumber, cabbage, carrots and green beans. Then transfer the vegetables to a colander and leave to drain in the sink for about 30 minutes, to allow excess water to drip away from the vegetables.

Grind the sesame seeds and peanuts into a fine powder using a pestle and mortar or food processor. Tip them out into a bowl.

Blitz the spice paste ingredients in a food processor or blender until they form a smooth paste.

Rinse the salt off the vegetables in the colander and set aside.

Set a wok or frying pan (skillet) over a medium heat. Add the coconut oil, wait for it to melt, then add the spice paste. Gently sauté for about 5 minutes until aromatic, then add the vinegar and water to the paste and leave to cook until it starts to boil. Add sugar to taste and turn off the heat. Add all the washed vegetables, the ground sesame seeds and the peanuts to the paste and stir well.

Let the pickle cool, then store it in a 1 litre (34 fl oz/ 4 cup) sterilised glass jar or container. You can eat it straight away, but *nyona acar* tastes better once the flavours have had a chance to develop (left at least overnight). The pickle will keep in the fridge for up to 1 month.

# ASIAN MAYO

*A velvety, creamy dream. This Asian mayo is perfect for coleslaws, summer salads and dipping. I keep a big tub in the fridge for times of flavoursome need.*

## Method

Put all the ingredients in a blender or food processor and blend on high speed until it's perfectly smooth. Its thick consistency makes it a great dipping sauce, but if you want to make a dressing then just add a little bit more water.

**Use this recipe to make:**
California Chirashi,
pg 88

### Ingredients

2 cm (¾ in) piece of fresh ginger root, rinsed and peeled

230 ml (7¾ fl oz/1 cup) olive oil

2 tsp sesame oil

juice of 1 lime

3 tbsp white miso paste

6 dates, pitted

2 tbsp soy sauce or tamari

80 ml (2¾ fl oz/⅓ cup) cold water

**Makes 1 big tub**

**Vegetarian**

**Vegan**

# BALANCING CHILLI OIL

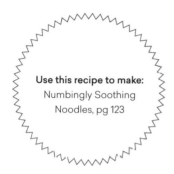

**Use this recipe to make:**
Numbingly Soothing
Noodles, pg 123

This oil is made with a blend of Chinese five-spice, Szechuan chilli and other spices. Five-spice actually refers to the five elements, not spices. According to traditional Chinese medicine, the five elements are manifested in different parts of the body and if there are imbalances in these elements, it causes disease. For thousands of years, different herbs and spices have been used to bring balance to the system and that is how five-spice powder came about.

This chilli oil is easy to make at home, packed with potent anti-inflammatory benefits, antioxidants and, above all, flavour. Szechuan peppercorns have a lemony, peppery, mouth-tingling tang to them. Drizzle this oil over cooked rice for an instant all-round boost to your system.

### Method

Combine all the spices (apart from the ginger, turmeric and oil) in a heatproof bowl that will hold at least 400 ml (14 fl oz/1¾ cups) liquid.

Heat the oil in a deep frying pan (skillet) over a medium-high heat, then add the ginger and turmeric matchsticks and fry for 3 minutes, or until the ginger starts to turn a golden brown colour. (You're aiming for the oil to reach a maximum of 190°C (375°F) if you have a thermometer to hand; otherwise, use the colour of your ginger to measure the oil temperature – when it turns golden, you're ready to pour.) Immediately turn off the heat.

Cautiously ladle or pour the hot oil into the bowl of mixed spices. The hot oil will bubble a little while it cooks the spices, but don't be alarmed. While it's bubbling, use a metal spoon to move them around, so they'll cook evenly. Leave to cool.

The longer the oil infuses, the tastier it will become. Store the oil in a sterilised airtight jar at room temperature. It will keep for up to 6 months.

*Recipe photo overleaf*

### Ingredients

4 tbsp dried Korean or Szechuan chilli (hot pepper) flakes

3 tbsp toasted white or black sesame seeds (or a mixture of both)

2 tsp Chinese five-spice powder

1 tsp Szechuan peppercorns

2 whole star anise

2 bay leaves

2 cm (¾ in) piece of fresh ginger root, peeled and cut into fine matchsticks

2 cm (¾ in) piece of fresh turmeric, peeled and cut fine matchsticks

240 ml (8½ fl oz/1 cup) olive oil (preferably light)

**Makes 260 ml (8¾ fl oz/ generous 1 cup)**

**Vegetarian**

**Vegan**

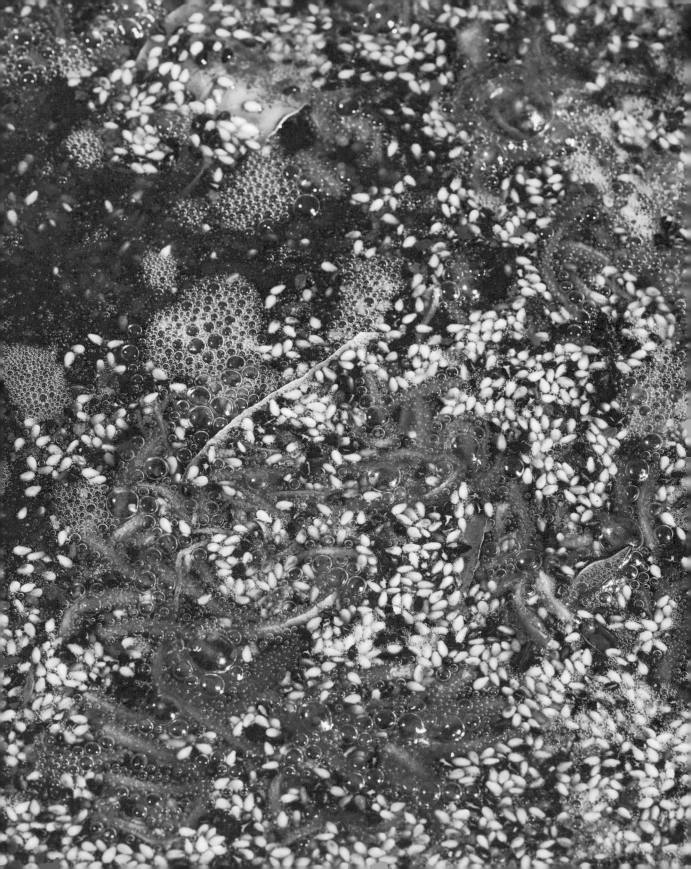

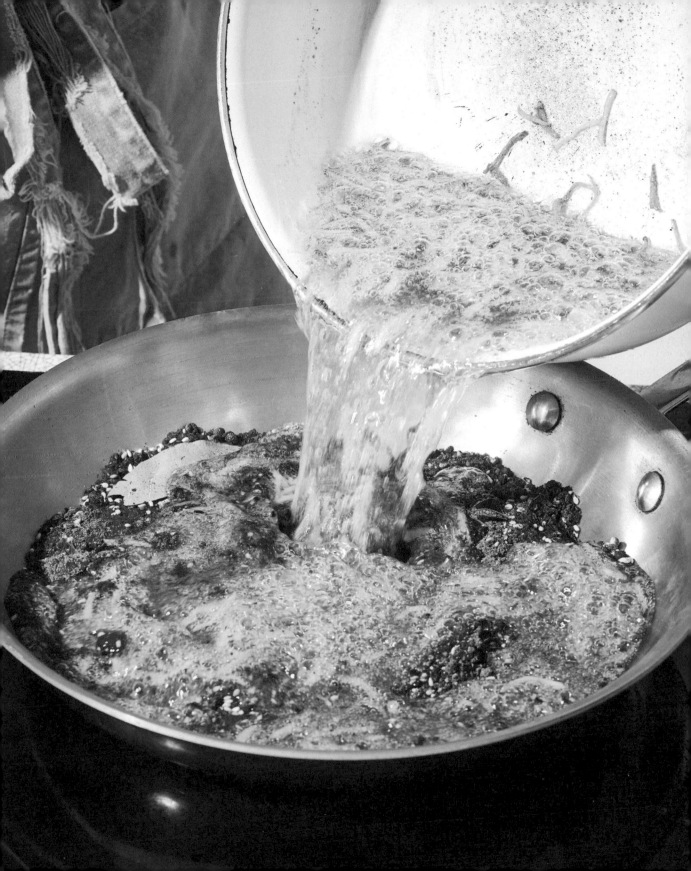

# EASY PROBIOTIC KIMCHI

## THE FUNKY KOREAN STAPLE

*Did you that know you can 'kimchi' just about anything? Kimchi-ing is a method for preserving vegetables – it's a verb. Before fridges were invented, different types of kimchi were traditionally made at different times of the year, based on the vegetables that were in season. This preserving method creates essential good bacteria and flavours that are mildly addictive. Don't limit yourself to cabbage – almost any seasonal vegetable will do.*

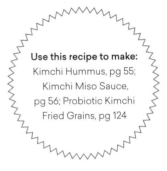

Use this recipe to make:
Kimchi Hummus, pg 55;
Kimchi Miso Sauce,
pg 56; Probiotic Kimchi
Fried Grains, pg 124

### Method

Put the sliced vegetables in a large bowl, add the water and the salt and toss well to mix them all up. The salt won't fully dissolve but it will still brine the vegetables. Leave at room temperature (uncovered) for about 2 hours.

Meanwhile, blitz all the 'kimchi anything' paste ingredients in a blender or food processor until smooth. Add a bit of water to loosen if necessary.

After you're done brining, drain the vegetables, rinse off all the salty water and gently squeeze the vegetables to remove excess water. Once thoroughly drained, put the vegetables in a bowl, add the paste and evenly massage the paste into the vegetables. Transfer the mixture to a 2 litre (70 fl oz/8 cup) plastic or glass container, seal and store in the fridge for up to a month, or longer if you like it fizzy. The longer you leave it to ferment, the more 'alive' the kimchi will become. The kimchi creates C02 gasses and will therefore start to fizz a little bit, but don't be alarmed – it's all just part of the fun.

### Ingredients

#### 'Kimchi Anything' Paste

5 garlic cloves

4 cm (1½ in) piece of fresh ginger root, peeled

80 g (3 oz) Korean chilli (hot pepper) flakes

50 ml (2 fl oz) fish sauce

5 anchovy fillets (tinned in oil)

2 tbsp unrefined sugar of choice

#### Vegetables

2 kg (4 lb 8 oz) any vegetable of choice, sliced

1 litre (34 fl oz/4 cups) filtered water

100 g (3½ oz) sea salt

**Makes 2 kg (4 lb 8 oz)**

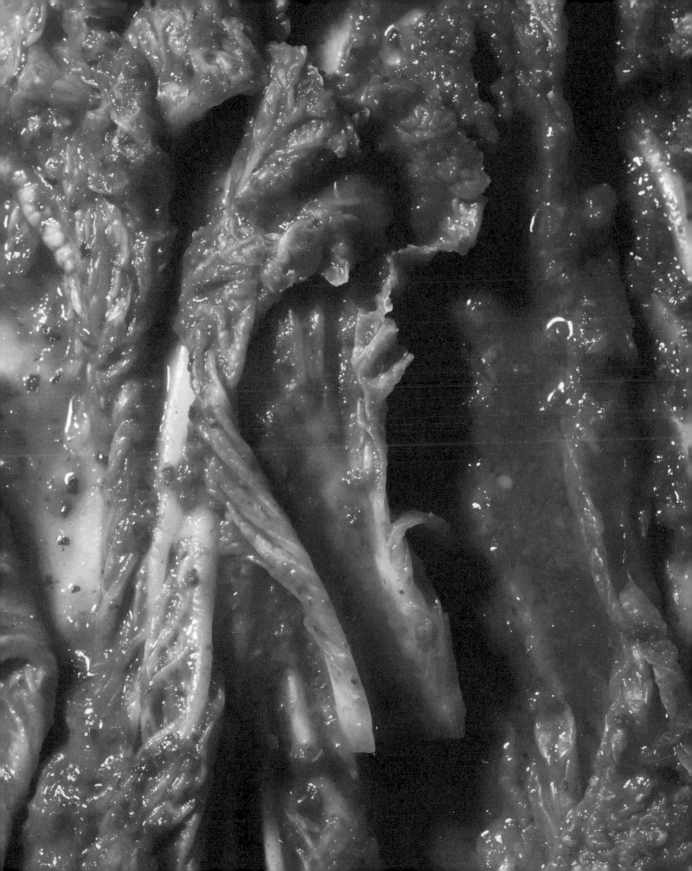

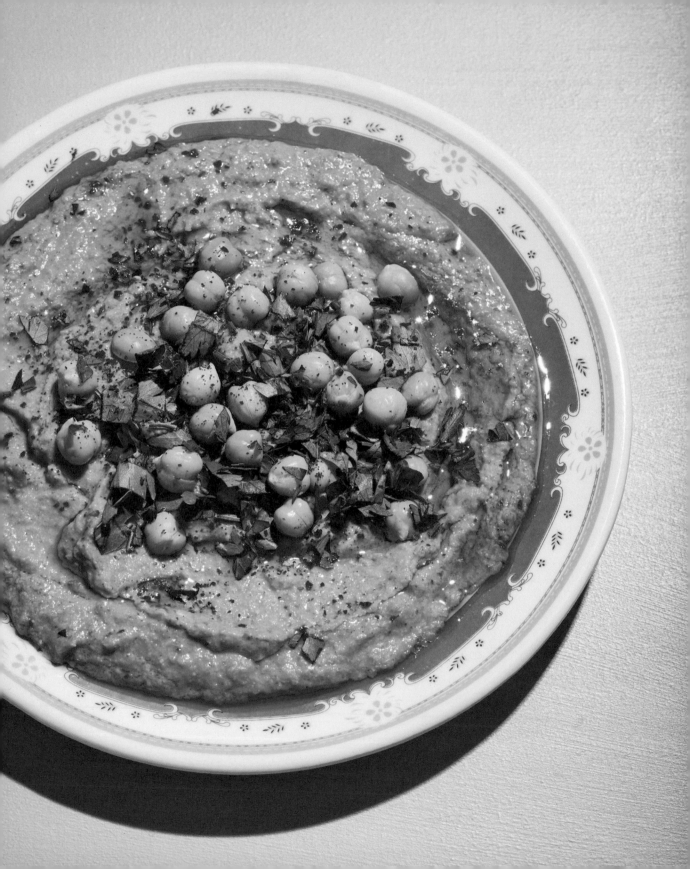

# KIMCHI HUMMUS

### Ingredients

400 g (14 oz) tin of chickpeas (garbanzos), rinsed

3 tbsp lemon juice

150 g (5 oz) Easy Probiotic Kimchi (page 52)

1 garlic clove

1 tbsp water

50 g (2 oz) tahini

100 ml (3½ fl oz/scant ½ cup) extra-virgin olive oil

½ tsp sesame oil

sea salt

**Makes about 450 g (1 lb)**

## SPICY & PROBIOTIC

*Amp up your hummus game with a Korean spin on this Middle Eastern classic. Spicy and sour, yet rich and creamy, this recipe combines two popular dishes from wildly different cultures, to make a spicy probiotic hummus. I sometimes reserve a few of the chickpeas and roast them for an added textural garnish. You can also top with chopped parsley when serving, for an extra flourish.*

### Method

Peel off the outer skin of each chickpea by rolling them between your fingers – it should come off really easily. This is vital for helping the digestion of these legumes as the skins are hard to digest and are what cause bloating.

Put all of the ingredients in a blender or food processor and blitz for about 2 minutes until the mixture is smooth and a pale red colour.

Scrape the hummus into a bowl and serve or store in the fridge in a sealed container for up to 2 weeks.

# KIMCHI MISO SAUCE

*This sauce makes an instant party in your mouth. Not only does it taste like Doritos, it's packed with fibre and potent probiotics too. Perfect for dunking crudités, corn chips or grilled cheese sandwiches into with your mates, or pouring over a salad or Bibimbap Wraps (page 118).*

## Ingredients

250 g (9 oz) Easy Probiotic Kimchi (page 52)

2 tbsp white miso paste

2 tbsp brown rice vinegar

60 ml (2 fl oz/¼ cup) olive oil

black and white sesame seeds, to serve

**Makes about 350 ml (12 fl oz/1½ cups)**

## Method

Put all of the ingredients (except for the sesame seeds) in a blender or food processor and blitz until smooth. Top with a sprinkling of sesame seeds when ready to serve. The sauce will keep in a sealed container in the fridge for up to 1 month.

# LEMONGRASS GUACAMOLE

*A zesty and invigorating twist on the classic avocado dip.*

## Ingredients

2 small garlic cloves

⅛ red onion

½ red chilli

1 lemongrass stalk, white part only

small bunch of coriander (cilantro)

2 large, ripe avocados

juice of ½ lime

sea salt and freshly ground black pepper

**Serves 2**

**Vegetarian**

**Vegan**

## Method

Put the garlic, red onion, chilli, lemongrass and coriander in a mortar and pound it with the pestle until smooth. Adding a pinch of sea salt will help to break down the ingredients.

Halve and stone one of the avocados and add the flesh to the mortar with the lime juice. Pound until partly smooth. Halve and stone the other avocado, add the flesh and pound just slightly, giving a bit of bite and texture to your guacamole. Season to taste with salt and pepper.

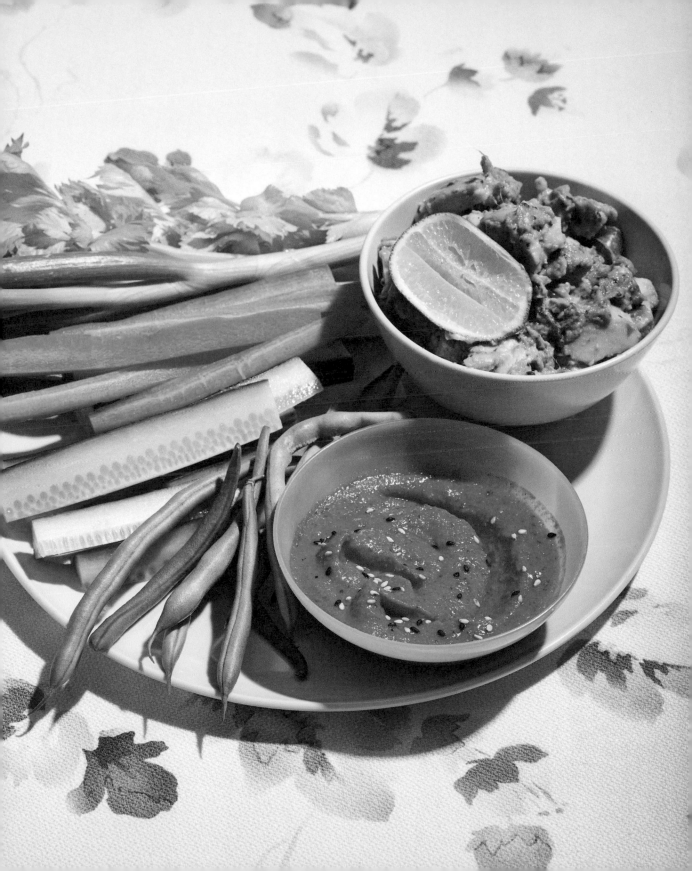

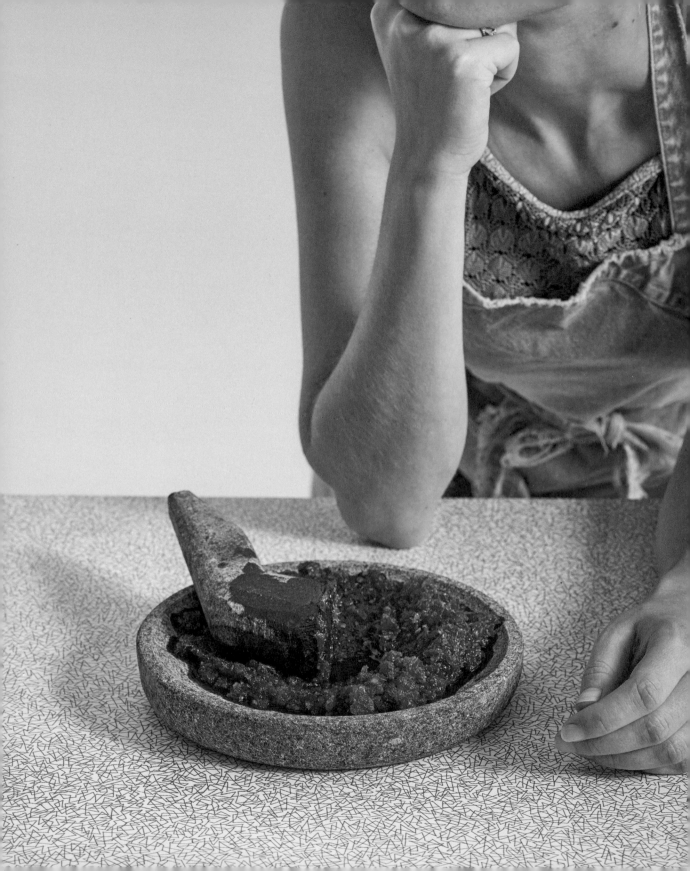

# GINGER & TOMATO SAMBAL

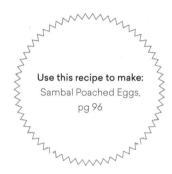

**Use this recipe to make:**
Sambal Poached Eggs,
pg 96

*This is not just any hot sauce, it is my favourite hot sauce. It is from Java, Indonesia, where it is known as* **sambal manis**. *Packed with ginger and garlic, it's a great sweet and spicy alternative to ketchup. Dollop this sambal on everything.*

## Ingredients

5 tomatoes, quartered

5 shallots

3 cm (1¼ in) piece of fresh ginger root

3 garlic cloves

2 anchovy fillets (tinned in oil) (optional)

8 red Thai chillies

4 tbsp coconut oil

3–4 tbsp coconut blossom nectar or unrefined caster (superfine) sugar

1 tsp sea salt, or to taste

**Makes about 200 g (7 oz)**

**To make this vegetarian or vegan, omit the anchovies, adding extra salt if needed**

## Method

Put the tomatoes, shallots, ginger, garlic, anchovies (if using) and chillies in a food processor or blender and pulse, adding a splash of water to help the process if needed, until you have a slightly textured paste. You're making a textured chutney, not a tomato passata, so don't over blend. This is traditionally made using a pestle and mortar, as photographed, so you are looking to mimic that course texture.

Now it's time to fry the paste: this will help develop its flavour. Place a wok or non-stick frying pan (skillet) over a high heat, then add the coconut oil. Once the oil has melted, add the paste. The paste contains water so be careful for any splash-back when you pour it in.

Stir the paste vigorously, reduce the heat to medium-high, and cook, stirring constantly, for 15–20 minutes, until the oil starts to separate from the paste and it develops a glossy texture.

At this stage, add the coconut blossom nectar, and the salt if needed, and turn off the heat. The sugar will caramelise so continue to stir, making sure to break up any clumps. Leave to cool to room temperature, then keep in a sealed container in the fridge for up to 2 weeks.

# LEMONGRASS & GINGER RELISH

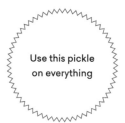

Use this pickle on everything

**Sambal matah** *comes from the heart of Bali. Slather the relish over freshly grilled fish like tuna, or on seafood, for a zingy and spicy anti-inflammatory, digestive aid and energy boost to the entire system. Instant summertime vibes.*

## Method

Combine all of the ingredients in a bowl and squeeze the mixture with your hands for about a minute to blend the flavours. Let it infuse for 10 minutes, then it's ready to serve. It's best used straight away, but will keep in the fridge for up to 24 hours.

## Ingredients

3 small green chillies, thinly sliced

8 small shallots, thinly sliced

2 lemongrass stalks, white part only, thinly sliced

2 cm (¾ in) piece of fresh ginger root, thinly sliced

pinch of sea salt

pinch of ground white pepper

3 tbsp coconut oil, melted

juice of ½ lime

1 kaffir lime leaf, thinly sliced (optional)

Serves 2

Vegetarian

Vegan

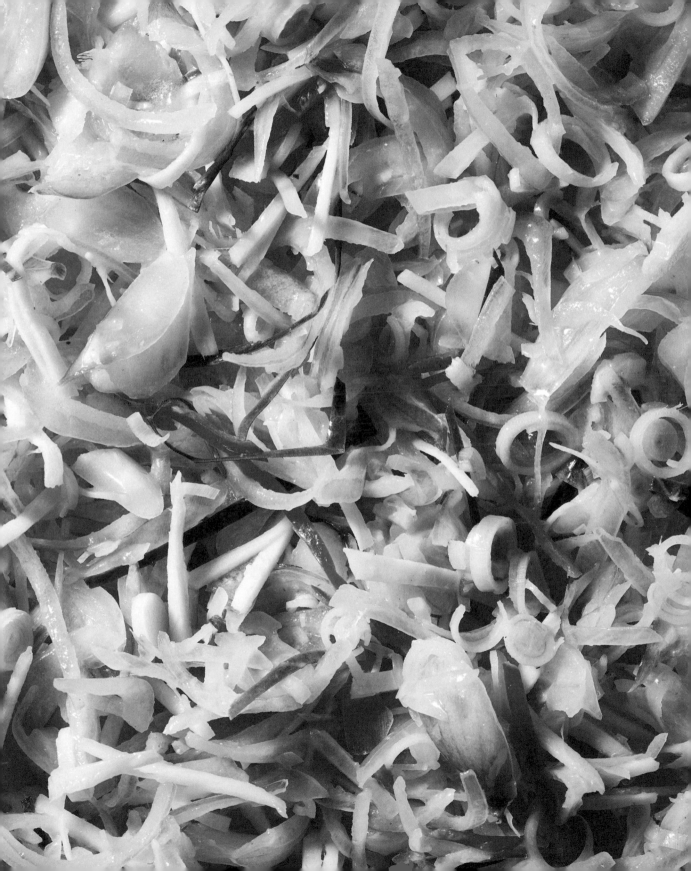

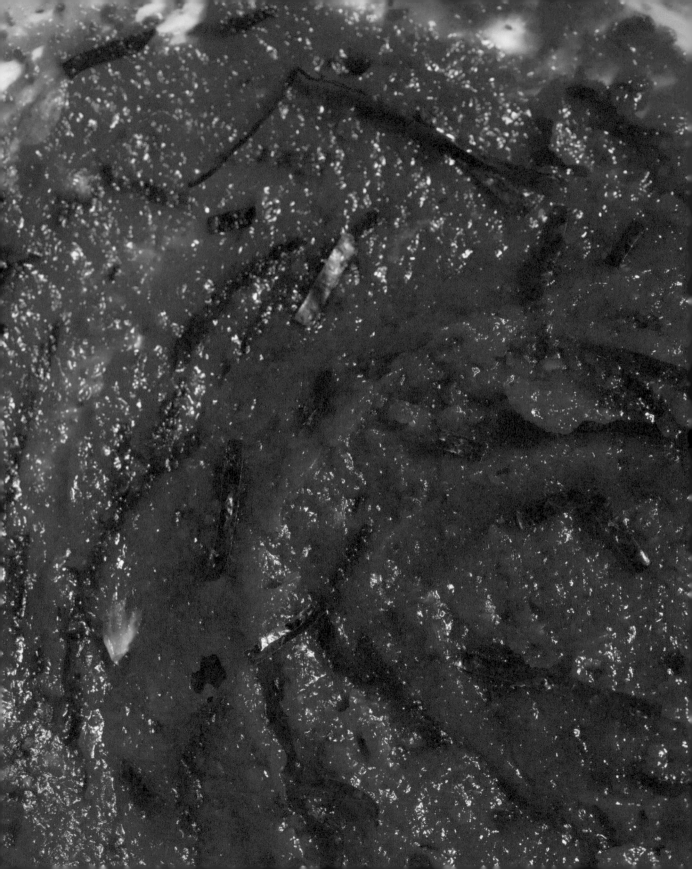

# GOCHUJANG

### Ingredients

2 tbsp white miso paste

2 tbsp Korean chilli (hot pepper) flakes (essential)

2 small garlic cloves, finely chopped

1 tbsp rice vinegar or apple cider vinegar

1 tbsp soy sauce, tamari or vegan liquid aminos

1 tsp sesame oil

1 tbsp honey or maple syrup

nori, cut into strips (optional)

**Use this recipe to make:**
Probiotic Kimchi
Fried Grains, pg 124;
Bibimbap Wraps, pg 118;
Korean Hangover Soup,
pg 106

**Makes about
50 g (2 oz)**

**Vegetarian**

**To make
this vegan,
substitute the
honey with
maple syrup**

**Gochujang** *is the bright red fermented paste found on your Bibimbap Wraps (page 118); it is the essence of Korean cooking. This is my easy 'cheat' recipe; equally tasty, and equally good for you. You can find miso and Korean chilli (hot pepper) flakes in all Asian supermarkets.*

### Method

Mix all the ingredients together and store in a sealed container in the fridge. It will keep for several weeks.

# INVIGORATING CURRY PASTE

## INSTANT BALI SUNSHINE IN YOUR MOUTH

*This curry paste, known as **bumbi bali**, captures the very essence of Balinese cuisine. It is the foundation of most recipes found on the island – packed with healing roots and spices. There's nothing more therapeutic than popping on some loud music, pouring a glass of wine, and smashing down a good curry paste in a pestle and mortar. Just saying.*

## Method

Depending on the day you've had, or how much time you have, pound all of the ingredients (apart from the oil, bay leaves and lemongrass) in a mortar with a pestle until you have a smooth paste. Alternatively, use a blender or food processor. You can add water to moisten the mixture. Don't worry if it gets too wet either, the moisture will evaporate during frying.

Heat the oil in a wok or heavy frying pan (skillet) over a medium-high heat, add the bay leaves and the lemongrass and cook for a minute or so. This will make the oil nice and fragrant. Then add the spice paste and cook for 10–15 minutes over a high heat, stirring frequently, until the mixture turns a rich golden brown colour and the oil starts to separate from the paste.

Remove from the heat and leave to cool before using. The cooled curry paste will keep in a sealed container in the fridge for up to 2 weeks, or a couple of months in the freezer (remove the bay leaves and lemongrass stalk first).

### Ingredients

10 tiny shallots or 2 white onions, peeled

4 garlic cloves

4 bird's eye chillies

5 cm (2 in) piece of fresh galangal (optional)

5 cm (2 in) piece of fresh ginger root

10 cm (4 in) piece of fresh turmeric

½ tbsp coriander seeds

6 candlenuts or blanched almonds

2 anchovy fillets (tinned in oil) (optional)

½ tsp ground nutmeg

1 tsp sea salt

1 tsp crushed white peppercorns

4 tbsp coconut oil

2 bay leaves

1 lemongrass stalk, bashed until it's pliable, and tied into a knot

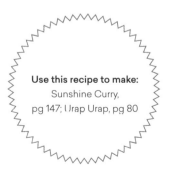

Use this recipe to make:
Sunshine Curry,
pg 147; Urap Urap, pg 80

Makes about
120 g (4 oz)

To make this vegetarian or vegan, omit the anchovies, adding extra salt if needed

# PROBIOTIC SRIRACHA

### Ingredients

500 g (1 lb 2 oz) red chillies (large serrano peppers are great)

1 tbsp sea salt

4 garlic cloves

1 tbsp fish sauce (optional)

3 tbsp sugar (palm sugar or unrefined cane sugar)

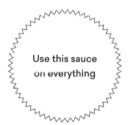

Use this sauce on everything

*This multi-purpose hot sauce is deliciously addictive. Not only do spicy peppers have amazing health benefits, traditional sriracha is actually fermented, and is therefore loaded with probiotic benefits too. This is the easiest fermented recipe I've ever made, and I've never looked back.*

### Method

Wash and wipe clean the chillies, then cut and discard the green ends. Put the chillies, salt, garlic and fish sauce (if using) in a blender or food processor and blitz until smooth.

Now it's time to ferment the sauce. Put the paste into a sterilised glass jar and seal the top with a muslin cloth. Store in a kitchen cupboard, away from direct sunlight, for 10–15 days (or longer if you prefer it a little funkier).

Once it is fermented, strain the paste through a sieve (fine-mesh strainer) into a saucepan. Add the sugar and cook over a medium heat for 1–2 minutes until it reaches the boil, then bottle in a sterilised glass jar. The bottled sriracha will keep for up to a year. Once opened, refrigerate to retain its freshness.

*Recipe photo overleaf*

**Makes 1 small jar (250 g/9 oz)**

**To make this vegetarian or vegan, omit the fish sauce, adding extra salt if needed**

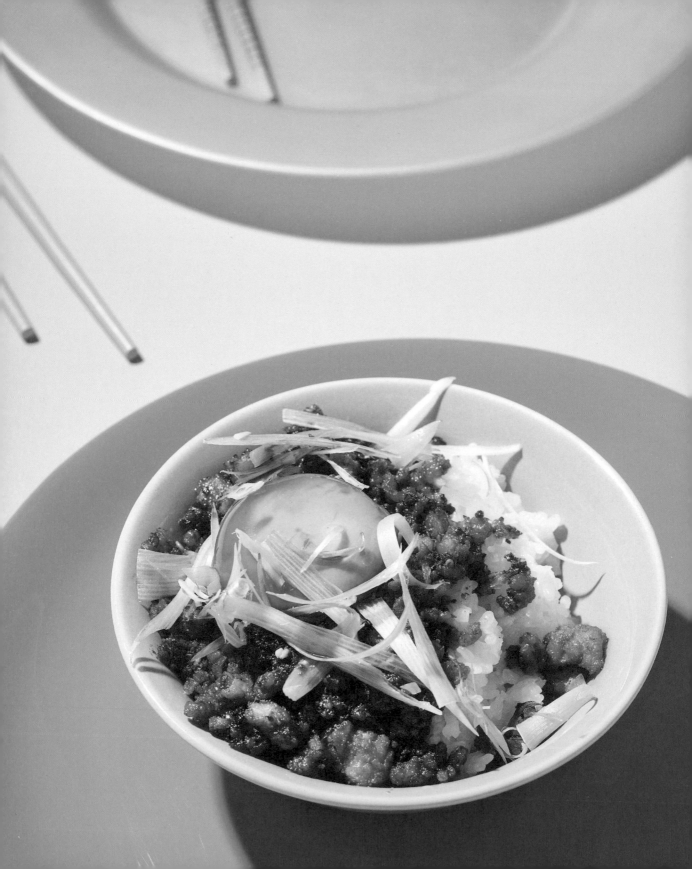

# SOY-CURED EGG YOLKS

## Ingredients

60 ml (2 fl oz/¼ cup) soy sauce
or tamari sauce

1 tbsp honey

2 cm (¾ in) piece of fresh
ginger root, finely chopped

4 eggs

Use these
soy-cured eggs
on everything

*When in doubt, put an egg on it. These salty,
oozy yolks are my go-to for instant flavour and
fermented goodness. It's like the Parmesan of
the East. Serve with pretty much anything –
it's great with a bowl of leftover rice.*

## Method

Put the soy or tamari sauce, honey and ginger
in a small bowl and whisk to combine.

Carefully separate the egg yolks from the whites,
then gently place the yolks in the soy sauce
mixture.

Cover the bowl of egg yolks and place in the fridge
to cure for 3–10 hours, swirling the bowl gently now
and again to make sure all the yolks are covered.
How long you leave them curing really depends
on how firm you like your yolk: you can cure them
for up to 2 days if liked. Add them onto a dish for
a cheesy and salty flavour. They are delicious.

**Makes 4
cured yolks**

**Vegetarian**

# TURMERIC PEANUT SAUCE

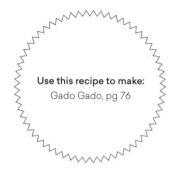

**Use this recipe to make:**
Gado Gado, pg 76

*Peanut sauce is the gateway to Indonesian food, and is also a staple condiment in every Dutch household. We put it on everything. Here's my supercharged ginger and turmeric version, for that extra boost.*

*To make this recipe, look for unsalted, unsweetened and roasted peanut butter. If you can't find it, roast your own peanuts (as photographed) and blend until smooth in a blender or food processor at home.*

## Method

Heat the coconut oil in a saucepan over a low–medium heat, then add the shallot, garlic, chilli, ginger, and turmeric. Sauté gently for 5 minutes, keeping the ingredients moving to stop them from colouring. Once they are glossy, add the peanut butter, kecap manis, coconut sugar, salt (to taste) and water to the pan and stir until fully combined and melted. Let the mixture simmer and thicken for about 5 minutes, stirring continuously, until it becomes a thick sauce. Turn off the heat and it's ready to serve.

The cooled sauce will keep in a sealed container in the fridge for up to 1 week. To reheat, simply add a splash of water and place back in a pan on the hob until you've reached the desired consistency again.

## Ingredients

1 tbsp coconut oil

1 shallot, finely diced

1 garlic clove, finely chopped

1 small bird's eye chilli, finely chopped

2 cm (¾ in) piece of fresh ginger root, grated

2 cm (¾ in) piece of fresh turmeric, grated

150 g (5 oz) peanut butter or roasted peanuts, blended to a butter

2 tbsp kecap manis (Indonesian sweet soy sauce)

1 tbsp coconut sugar

150 ml (5 fl oz/scant ⅔ cup) water

sea salt, to taste (about 1 tbsp)

Serves 4

Vegetarian

Vegan

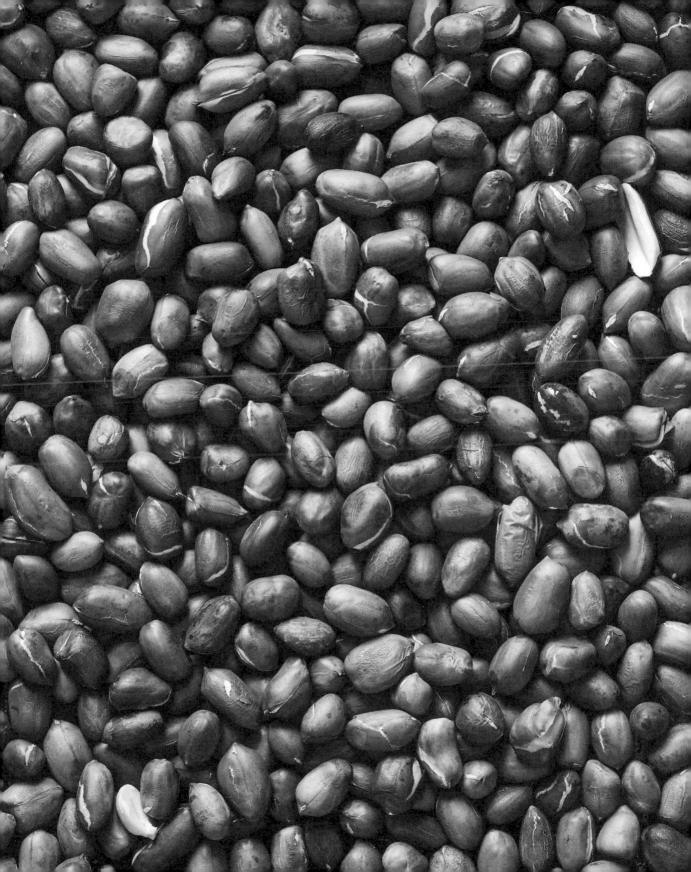

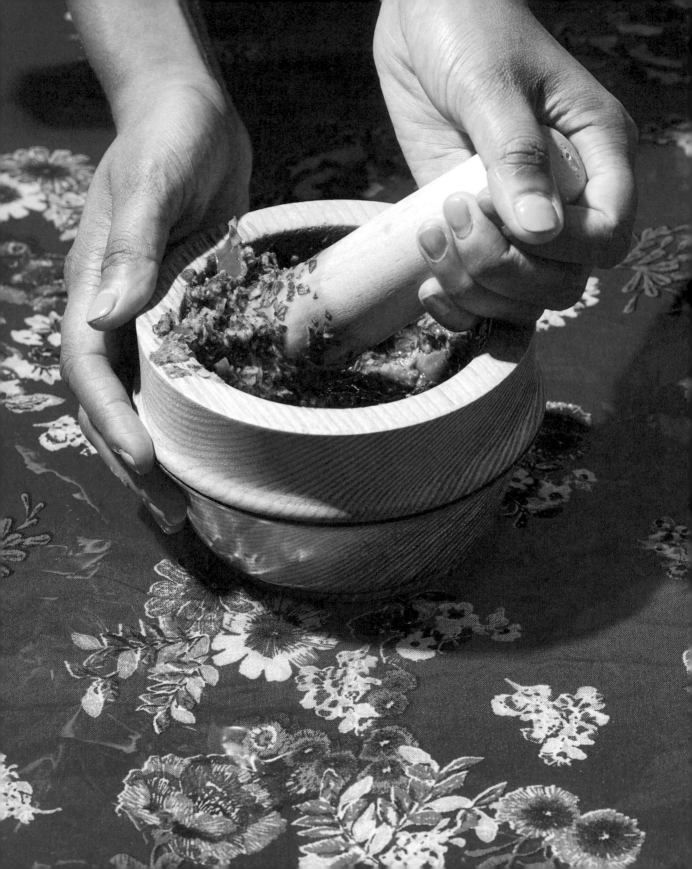

# SPICED SALSA VERDE

## Ingredients

seeds from 2 green cardamom pods

1 tsp black peppercorns

1 tsp coriander seeds

½ tsp cumin seeds

4 green jalapeño chillies

2 garlic cloves

4 anchovy fillets (tinned in oil) (optional)

large pinch of sea salt

generous handful of parsley leaves, finely chopped

generous handful of coriander (cilantro) leaves, finely chopped

100 ml (3½ fl oz/scant ½ cup) olive oil

juice of 1 lemon

Makes about 140 g (5 oz)

To make this vegetarian or vegan, omit the anchovies, adding extra salt if needed

**Use this salsa to serve with:**
Lemongrass Rendang, pg 82

*Zhoug is Yemen's answer to salsa verde, or pesto. This sauce is fresh, fiery, exciting and packed with pungent and soothing herbs and spices. Yemenites swear by its health benefits and eat it daily to deliciously enhance their wellbeing.*

## Method

Toast the cardamom seeds, peppercorns, coriander seeds and cumin seeds in a small dry frying pan (skillet) over a medium-high heat for a few minutes until fragrant. Tip them into a mortar then grind to a fine powder with a pestle and leave to cool.

Add the chillies, garlic and anchovy fillets (if using) to the mortar, sprinkle with a large pinch of salt and smash to make a paste.

Add the herbs and oil and work them into the mixture with the pestle. Leave the spiced salsa verde to sit and infuse for 10 minutes, then finish with the lemon juice. Use straight away.

TIRED?

FIGHT FATIGUE BY EATING WELL. WHAT YOU EAT CAN HAVE A HUGE IMPACT ON YOUR ENERGY LEVELS. IF YOU'RE LOOKING FOR WAYS TO PERK YOURSELF UP, TRY THESE SPICED RECIPES AT HOME. THE INGREDIENTS WILL HELP GIVE YOUR BODY THE BOOST IT NEEDS, AND MAKE YOU FEEL MORE ENERGISED AND INVIGORATED THAN EVER.

# GADO GADO

*The most nostalgically 'Dutch' meal I know is in fact Indonesian street food. **Gado gado** means 'mix mix' and you essentially mix everything up and tuck in. It's also how you colloquially refer to people from mixed cultural backgrounds in Bahasa, hence the sentimental value here. Packed full of energising veggies, spices and legumes, the combination of textures and flavours make this salad both satisfying and invigorating. Use any seasonal vegetables of choice. I serve this with the Turmeric Peanut Sauce (page 70), prawn crackers and a steamed egg. Cooked rice is great, too.*

## Method

Put the potatoes in a pan of water, bring to the boil and cook until soft.

Meanwhile, cook the green beans in a saucepan of salted boiling water for 2 minutes, then add the softer vegetables (cabbage, spinach and bean sprouts) and cook for another minute. Drain, rinse under cold running water and leave in a colander, squeezing off the excess water every couple of minutes with your hands.

Melt the coconut oil in a deep frying pan (skillet) over a medium-high heat until it reaches 160–180ºC (320–350ºF) (if you don't have a thermometer, put a wooden spoon in the oil – as soon as bubbles start to come to the surface, the oil is ready). Fry the tempeh and tofu (if using) in batches, separately, for 5 minutes each until golden brown all over and the tempeh is crispy.

Place all the cooked vegetables on a large serving dish with the tofu and tempeh. Then, slather the peanut sauce over them generously (if using). You can use a pestle and mortar to help mix everything up.

Serve, with the eggs and crackers.

## Ingredients

150 g (5 oz) new potatoes, halved

handful of green beans, trimmed and each cut into 3 pieces

¼ cabbage of choice, thinly sliced

200 g (7 oz) spinach

200 g (7 oz) bean sprouts

8–10 tbsp coconut oil

50 g (2 oz) tempeh, thinly sliced (optional)

50 g (2 oz) firm tofu, thinly sliced (optional)

Turmeric Peanut Sauce (page 70) (optional)

## To Serve

2 eggs, steamed for 7 minutes (see Cook's Notes on page 19), then peeled and halved. (optional)

prawn crackers (optional)

**Serves 2–3**

**To make this vegetarian or vegan, omit the crackers and eggs**

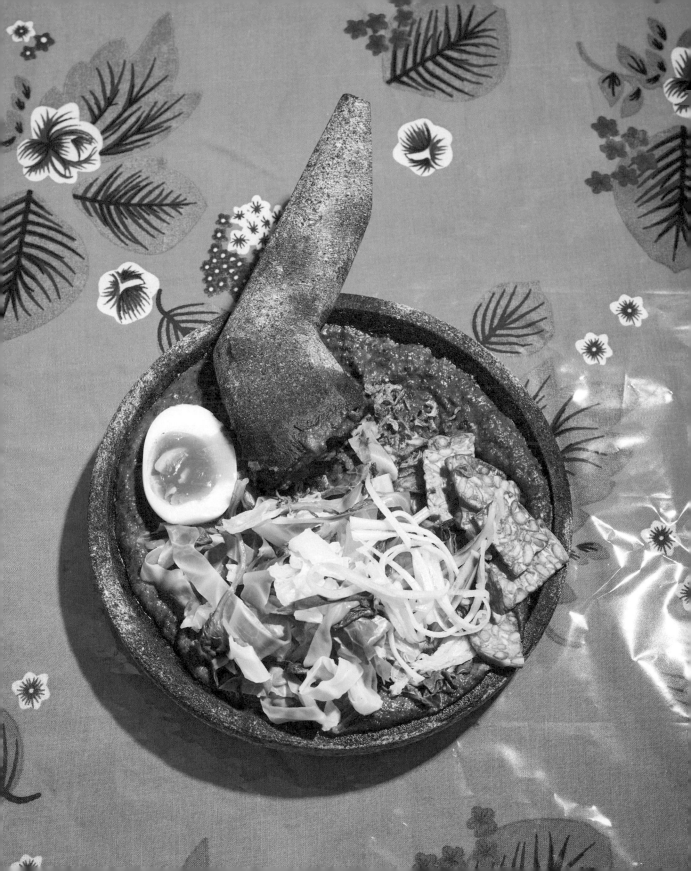

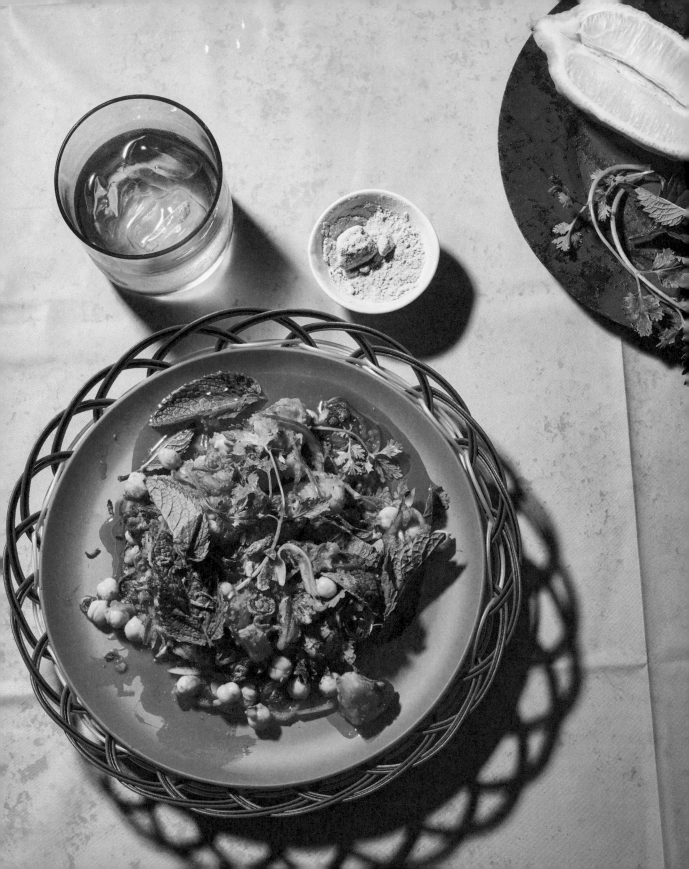

# SWEET POTATO CHAAT

### Ingredients

3 large sweet potatoes or yams, peeled

2 tbsp tamarind water (see Cook's Notes on page 20) or 1 tbsp tamarind concentrate

juice of 2 limes

1 tbsp honey or maple syrup

1 tsp dried chilli (hot pepper) flakes

1 tsp cumin seeds, toasted

1 tsp chaat masala

1 red onion, thinly sliced

400 g (14 oz) tin of chickpeas (garbanzos), rinsed

1 tomato, chopped

handful of coriander (cilantro), roughly chopped

handful of mint leaves

olive oil, for drizzling

black salt or sea salt, to taste

**Serves 4**

**Vegetarian**

**To make this vegan, substitute the honey with maple syrup**

*Chaat is a street food snack from Delhi, India, and chaat masala is a very popular spice blend from northern India that you can find in most Asian supermarkets. It's a wonderfully spicy, sour and salty blend that complements the sweetness of the energising potatoes, chickpeas and quick-pickled onion deliciously. Instead of the usual potato, I've used comforting sweet potatoes. Yams work just as well.*

### Method

Cook the sweet potatoes or yams in a saucepan of boiling salted water until tender, then drain.

Combine the tamarind water, lime juice, honey or maple syrup, chilli flakes, cumin seeds and chaat masala in a large salad bowl. Mix well and stir in the sliced onion. Leave it to pickle.

Once your sweet potatoes or yams have cooled slightly, chop them into bite-sized chunks and add them to the onion and zingy dressing.

Peel off the outer skin of each chickpea by rolling each of them between the fingers – it should come off really easily. This is vital for helping the digestion of these legumes as the skins are hard to digest and are what cause bloating. Add the chickpeas to the salad bowl along with the chopped tomato and fresh coriander, mint and salt to taste. Drizzle with a fair glug of olive oil (don't be shy!).

# URAP URAP

### Ingredients

50 g (2 oz) green beans, trimmed and cut into 3 cm (1¼ in) lengths

100 g (3½ oz) carrots, cut into 3 cm (1¼ in) chunks

100 g (3½ oz) cabbage of choice, cut into 3 cm (1¼ in) chunks

100 g (3½ oz) spinach

100 g (3½ oz) bean sprouts

2 tbsp Invigorating Curry Paste (page 64)

200 g (7 oz) freshly grated coconut (about 1 whole coconut)

100 ml (3½ fl oz/scant ½ cup) tamarind pulp, soaked in warm water and strained (see Cook's Note on page 20) (optional)

juice of 1 lime, or to taste

sea salt, to taste

## BALI-SPICED COCONUT SALAD

*This crunchy Indonesian salad is made with a potent anti-inflammatory curry paste and packed with deliciously sweet freshly grated coconut.*

### Method

Cook the green beans and carrots in a saucepan of salted boiling water for 2 minutes, then add the softer vegetables (cabbage, spinach and bean sprouts) and cook for another minute. Drain, rinse under cold running water and leave in a colander, squeezing off the excess water every couple of minutes with your hands.

In a large mixing bowl, mix the spice paste with the freshly grated coconut using your fingers, then slowly start to add the blanched vegetables, until everything is well coated and combined.

Add the strained tamarind liquid, sea salt and lime juice to the bowl, to taste. Mix together then serve.

### Serves 4

To make this vegetarian or vegan, omit the anchovies from the curry paste, adding extra salt if needed

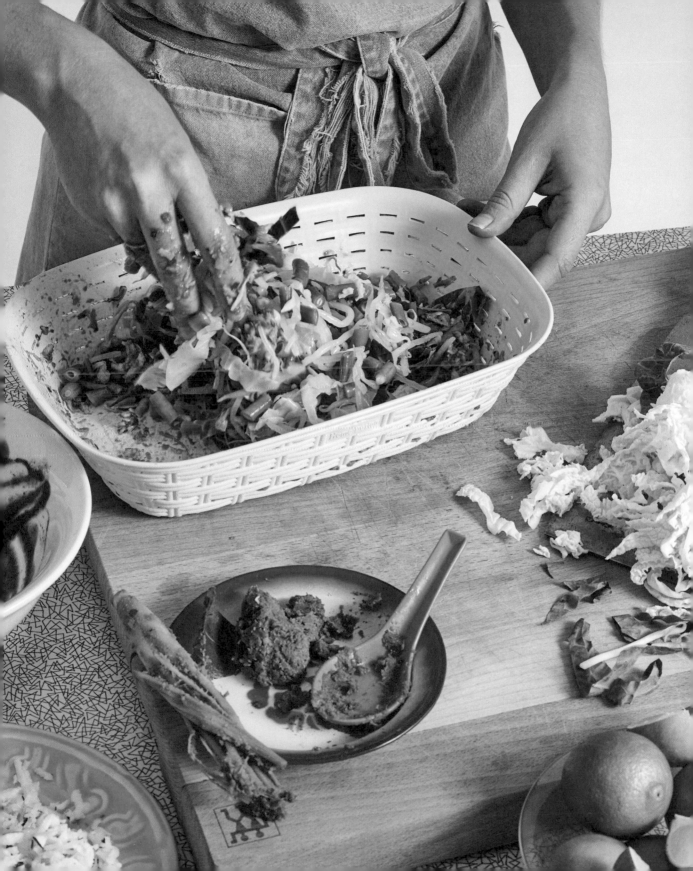

# LEMONGRASS RENDANG

## Ingredients

### Spice Paste

5 small shallots, peeled and roughly chopped

2 cm (¾ in) piece of fresh ginger root, peeled and roughly chopped

2 cm (¾ in) piece of fresh turmeric, roughly chopped

2 cm (¾ in) piece of fresh galangal, peeled and roughly chopped (optional)

3 lemongrass stalks, white part only, roughly chopped

4 candlenuts or blanched almonds, roughly chopped

5 garlic cloves, roughly chopped

3 green bird's eye chillies, roughly chopped

### Rendang

5 tbsp coconut oil

1 cinnamon stick

1 tsp ground coriander

3 cloves

3 star anise

2 bay leaves

seeds from 3 green cardamom pods, crushed

1 kg (2 lb 4 oz) beef short ribs, stewing beef (cubed) or jackfruit

1 lemongrass stalk, bruised

400 ml (14 fl oz) tin of coconut milk

2 tbsp fresh tamarind water (see Cook's Note on page 20) or 1 tbsp tamarind concentrate

400 ml (14 fl oz/1¾ cups) water

6 tbsp grated coconut, freshly toasted

1 tbsp coconut palm sugar, or more to taste

sea salt

### To Serve

12 corn tacos, Spiced Salsa Verde (page 73), coconut yoghurt and lime wedges **or** boiled jasmin rice, fried eggs, coriander (cilantro)

### Serves 4

**To make this vegetarian, substitute the beef with jackfruit**

## Method

Put all the spice paste ingredients in a blender or food processor and blitz to a smooth spice paste.

To make the rendang, heat the coconut oil in a large casserole dish (Dutch oven), add the spice paste, cinnamon stick, ground coriander, cloves, star anise, bay leaves and crushed cardamom and fry, stirring constantly, for 10 minutes until aromatic.

Add the beef (or jackfruit) and pounded lemongrass and stir for 1 minute, then add the coconut milk, tamarind water (or concentrate) and water, and cook over a medium heat, stirring frequently, until it comes back up to the boil.

Add the toasted coconut and coconut sugar, then reduce the heat to low, part cover with a lid and simmer for 2–3 hours until the sauce has thickened, and starts drying up. The meat should be soft and tender (falling off the bone, if you've used beef ribs). Check it every 30 minutes or so, stirring the sauce to make sure nothing sticks to the bottom. If you're using jackfruit instead of beef, cook the curry for no longer than an hour. The consistency will be saucier, but that's delicious too.

Add salt and more coconut sugar to taste, if needed. Serve either with the tacos, coconut yoghurt, lime-pickled onions, lime wedges and salsa verde, or with rice, a fried egg and coriander.

*Recipe photos overleaf*

## RENDANG IS ALWAYS BETTER THE NEXT DAY

*This is a festive dish made for sharing by the people of West Sumatra, Indonesia. It's simmered for a long time, which allows the meat to soak up all of the spices, resulting in a dry aromatic beef curry. Although this recipe calls for a lot of roots, herb and spices, don't let that put you off; they are packed with antimicrobial properties and, above all, flavour – making this recipe well worth your time. Serve it on corn tacos, or on rice with a fried egg the next day. (Both are pictured on the next page.)*

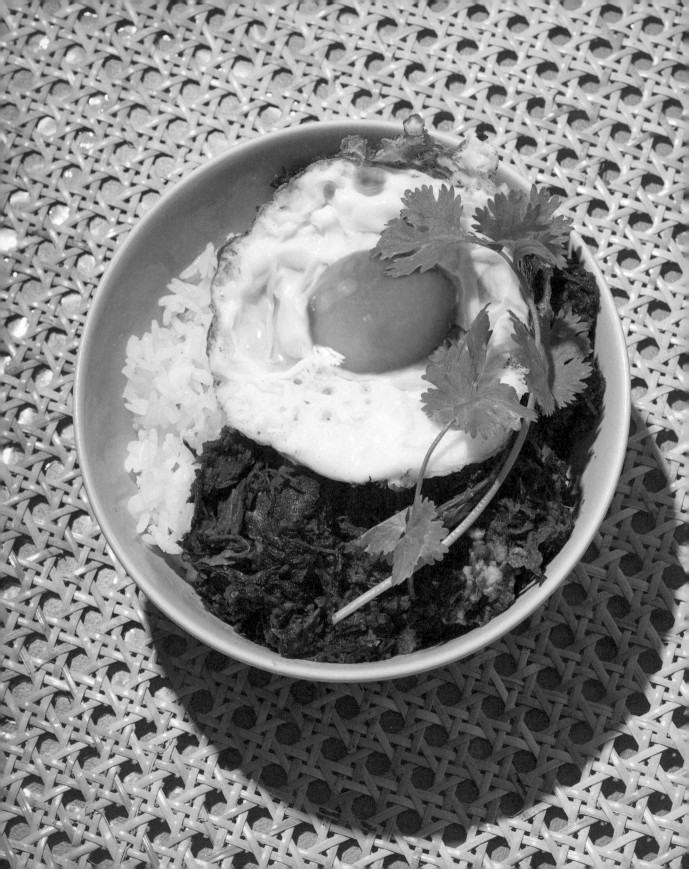

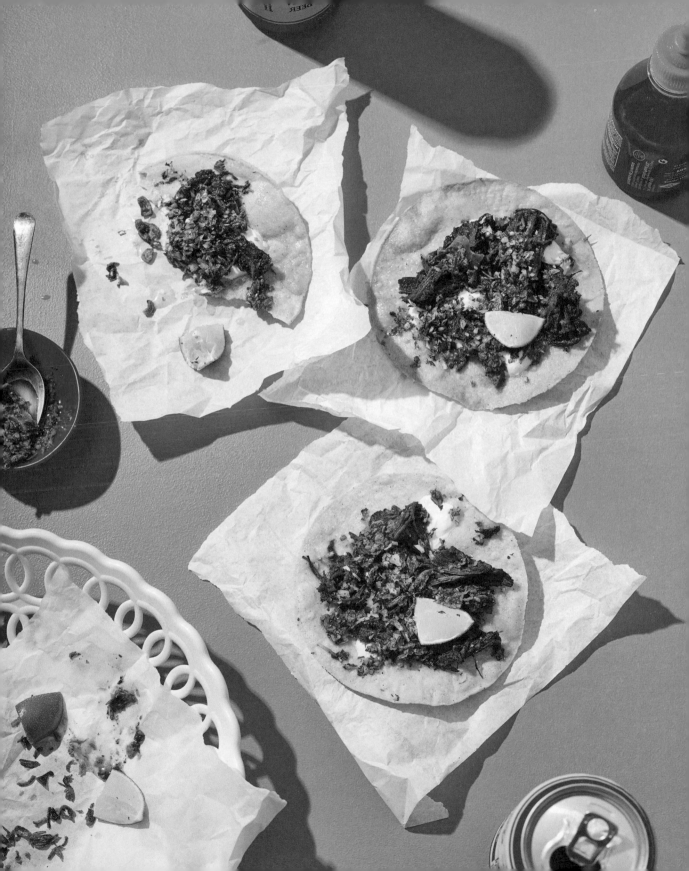

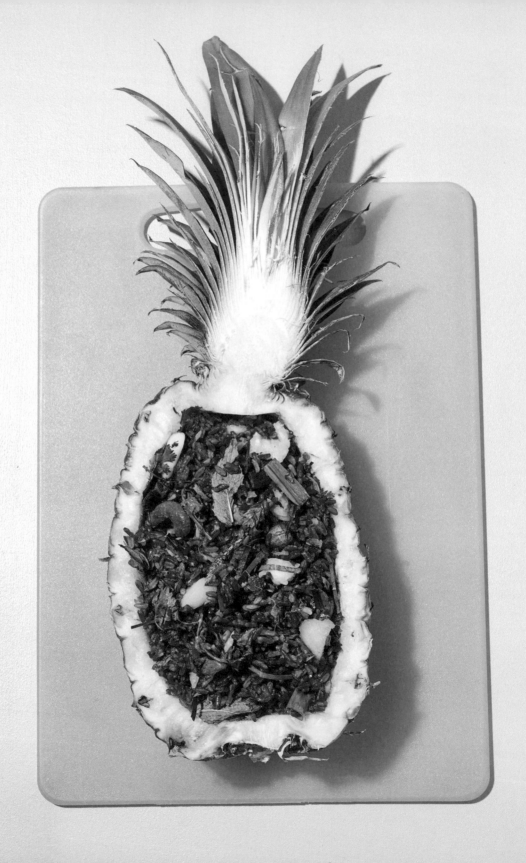

# TOM YUM
# FRIED RICE

## Ingredients

1 tbsp coconut oil

1 lemongrass stalk, white part only, thinly sliced

2 cm (¾ in) piece of fresh ginger root, peeled and grated

1 shallot, thinly sliced

2 garlic cloves, finely chopped

2 small red Thai chillies, thinly sliced

100 g (3½ oz) pineapple, finely chopped

300 g (10½ oz) cooked rice of your choice or 180 g (6 oz) uncooked rice

1 tbsp fish sauce

2 tbsp kecap manis (Indonesian sweet soy sauce)

100 g (3½ oz/⅔ cup) roasted cashews

1 kaffir lime leaf, thinly sliced (optional)

1 lime, halved

**Serves 2**

**To make this vegetarian, omit the fish sauce, adding extra salt if needed**

*Spicy, savoury and a little sour, this tangy fried rice is packed with the energising and invigorating flavours of Thai Tom Yum. I like to use nutty red rice for this recipe, but any leftover rice will work just fine.*

## Method

Heat a wok or large frying pan (skillet) over a high heat, add the coconut oil, then add the lemongrass, ginger, shallot, garlic and chillies. Sauté for about 6 minutes, stirring constantly to prevent the ingredients from colouring. Add the pineapple and the cooked rice to the sizzling wok and mix everything together. Reduce the heat to medium, add the fish sauce, kecap manis, cashews and kaffir lime leaf (if liked). Stir and fry for 2–3 minutes until the rice is hot and steamy.

Turn off the heat and finish with a squeeze of lime juice.

# CALIFORNIA CHIRASHI

*Inspired by Japanese chirashi bowls and California rolls, this is a very convenient way of making 'sushi' at home. The word **'chirashi'** means 'scattered', and usually consists of a few varieties of sashimi scattered over some rice.*

*Chirashi originated in the Edo period (1603–1868). It's a dish that the commoners made for special occasions. During this time, the government strictly monitored all social order, and would not condone any extravaganzas when it came to expenditures, so when people made chirashi, they would hide all the toppings on the bottom of the large plate, and cover them with rice. When it was time to eat and celebrate, they would simply flip the dish over and tuck in. Brilliant.*

*Every family has their own humble version of chirashi at home in Japan. It's never fancy, but always comforting. California rolls were my favourite as a kid, so this topping feels very nostalgic and appropriate to me. With this, I hope their legacy rolls on.*

## Method

Cook the rice according to the packet instructions. Once cooked, allow it to cool.

Mix the crab meat (if using) into the Asian or regular mayo, then layer all of the ingredients on top of two bowls of the cooled rice. Pour some soy sauce or tamari over the top and sprinkle on some togarashi, if you wish. Mix up all the ingredients and enjoy.

## Ingredients

180 g (6 oz/generous ¾ cup) short-grain brown or white rice

200 g (7 oz) crab meat (white and brown) (optional)

6 tbsp Asian Mayo (page 48) or regular mayonnaise

1 ripe avocado, halved, stoned and chopped into cubes

½ long cucumber, julienned

1 spring onion (scallion), trimmed and thinly sliced

2 sheets of toasted nori, shredded

2 tbsp toasted sesame seeds (white or black)

Korean Turmeric Pickle (page 44) (optional), finely sliced

soy sauce or tamari, to serve (optional)

shichimi togarashi, to serve (optional)

**Serves 2**

**To make this vegetarian, omit the crab meat**

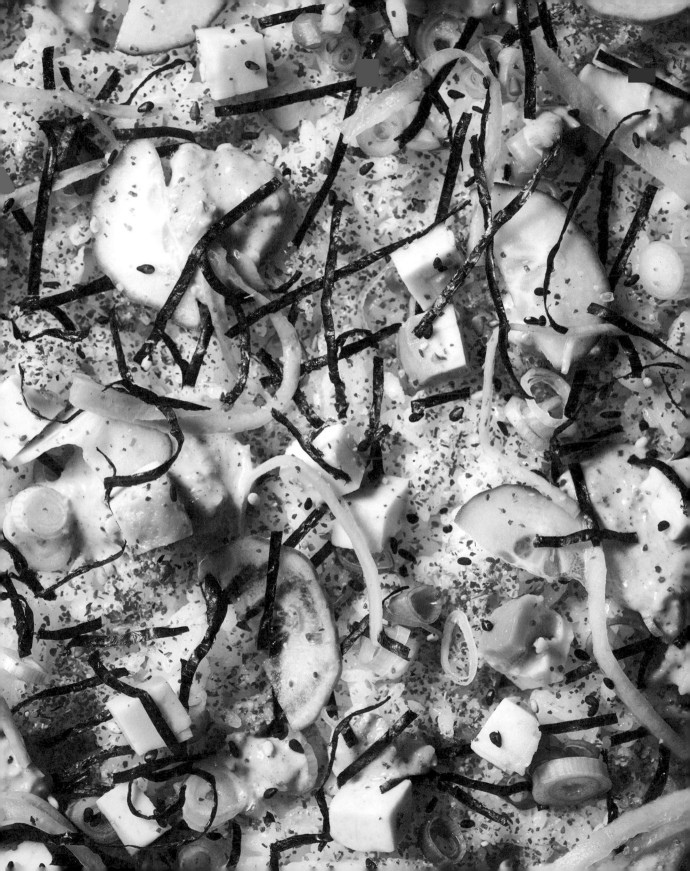

# HUNGOVER?

ONLY A TRUE BON VIVANT IS EQUIPPED TO CURE A HANGOVER WITH FOOD ALONE. THIS CHAPTER'S GOT YOU COVERED WITH RELIABLE REMEDIES PACKED WITH EGG YOLKS, SPICE & ANTI-INFLAMMATORY GOODNESS.

# RUJAK

*This traditional Indonesian fruit salad is a scrumptious mix of spicy, sweet, salty, tangy and crunchy flavours and textures that aim to pick you up and cool you down.*

## Method

Start by making the spicy peanut dressing: put the tamarind liquid in a pestle and mortar with the rest of the dressing ingredients (using just half the peanuts) and pound until you have a smooth sauce. Crush the remaining peanuts lightly for sprinkling over the finished dish.

Put the fruit in two bowls or a large serving platter and pour over the dressing. Sprinkle with the crushed peanuts and serve with lime 'cheeks'.

### Ingredients

½ pineapple, peeled and cut into chunks

2 cucumbers, peeled and cut into chunks

1 eating (dessert) apple, cored and sliced (I prefer to leave the skin on)

2 'cheeks' of lime, dipped in salt and dried chilli (hot pepper) flakes

### Spicy Peanut Dressing

20 g (¾ oz) tamarind pulp, soaked in warm water and strained (see Cook's Note on page 36)

100 ml (3½ fl oz/scant ½ cup) warm water

100 g (3½ oz) coconut palm sugar

1 red chilli

1 tsp grated fresh ginger root

1 tsp sea salt

juice of ½ lime

2 tbsp coconut sugar

100 g (3½ oz/scant ⅔ cup) roasted peanuts

Serves 2

Vegetarian

Vegan

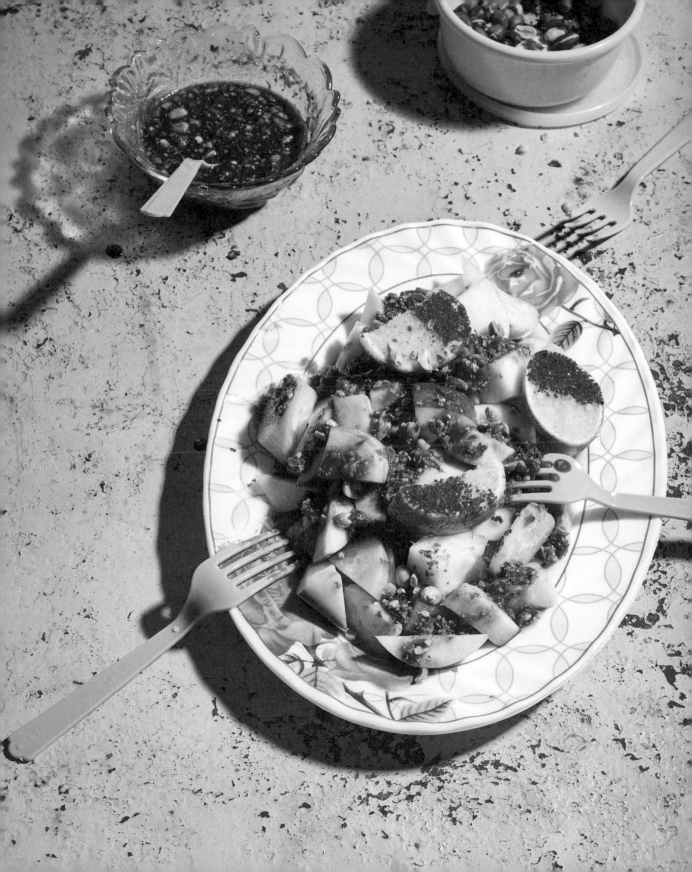

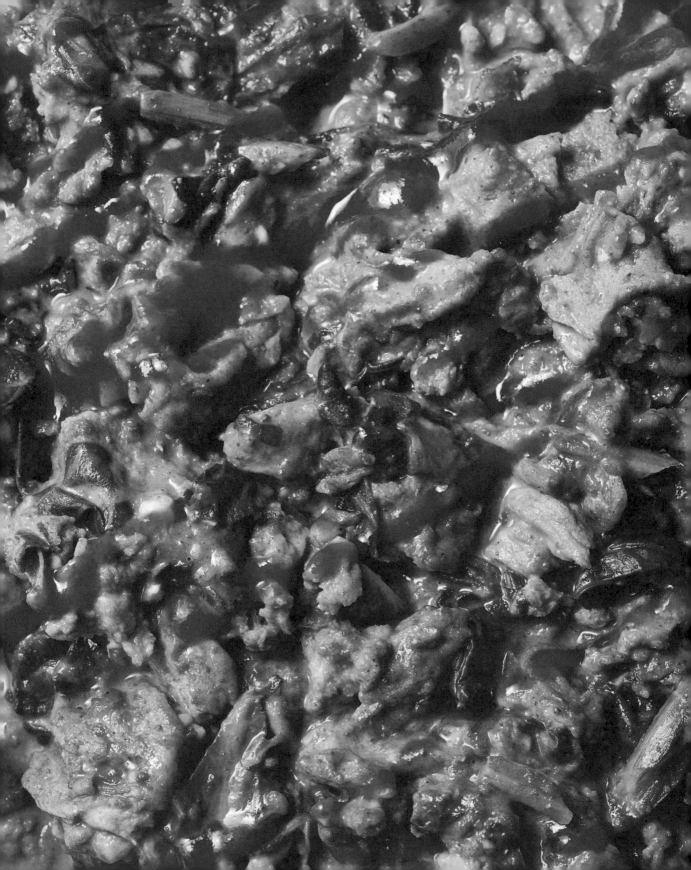

# TURMERIC SCRAMBLED EGGS

## Ingredients

4 eggs

50 ml (2 fl oz/3 tbsp) coconut milk

2 cm (¾ in) piece of fresh turmeric, grated, or 2 tsp ground turmeric

2 tbsp coconut oil

1 garlic clove, finely chopped

2 generous handfuls of spinach

sea salt and freshly ground black pepper

## To Serve

sourdough bread, toasted

Probiotic Sriracha (page 65) or shop-bought, for drizzling

*These anti-inflammatory scrambled eggs will mop up any toxins from the night before.*

## Method

Whisk the eggs in a bowl or jug with the coconut milk and ground turmeric. Season well with salt and pepper.

Melt the coconut oil in a non-stick frying pan (skillet) over a medium heat. Add the garlic and fry for 2 minutes, then add the spinach and cook briefly until it wilts.

Add the egg mixture to the garlic and spinach. Then stir continuously until the scrambled eggs are at the desired consistency.

Serve the turmeric scrambled eggs on toasted sourdough bread and drizzle with some sriracha.

Serves 2

Vegetarian

# SAMBAL POACHED EGGS

## Ingredients

2 tbsp coconut oil

2 tbsp Ginger & Tomato Sambal (page 59)

400 g (14 oz) tin of coconut milk

2 eggs

sea salt, to taste

small bunch of coriander (cilantro), chopped

juice of 1 lime

crispy shallots, to serve (optional)

*The best hangover cures come poached and sunny side up. This is an Indonesian-style take on the classic shakshuka, made with ginger and tomato sambal and coconut milk. Ginger is a well-known treatment for nausea – perfect for when your stomach is churning and you're feeling queasy.*

*Serve these poached eggs with crusty bread or roti for dipping, or a side of steamed rice.*

## Method

Heat the coconut oil in a non-stick frying pan (skillet) over a medium heat then add the ginger and tomato sambal and fry until aromatic. Stir in the coconut milk and let it simmer for about 3 minutes.

Carefully crack the eggs into the pan, cover with a lid and cook until the egg whites are set and the yolks are still runny (this may take up to 10 minutes). Season with salt.

Toss the coriander in the lime juice then sprinkle it over the eggs. Bring to the table in the pan with a sprinkle of crispy shallots (if using), to serve over rice or mop up with cruchy bread or roti.

**Serves 2**

**To make this vegetarian, omit the anchovies from the sambal, adding extra salt if needed**

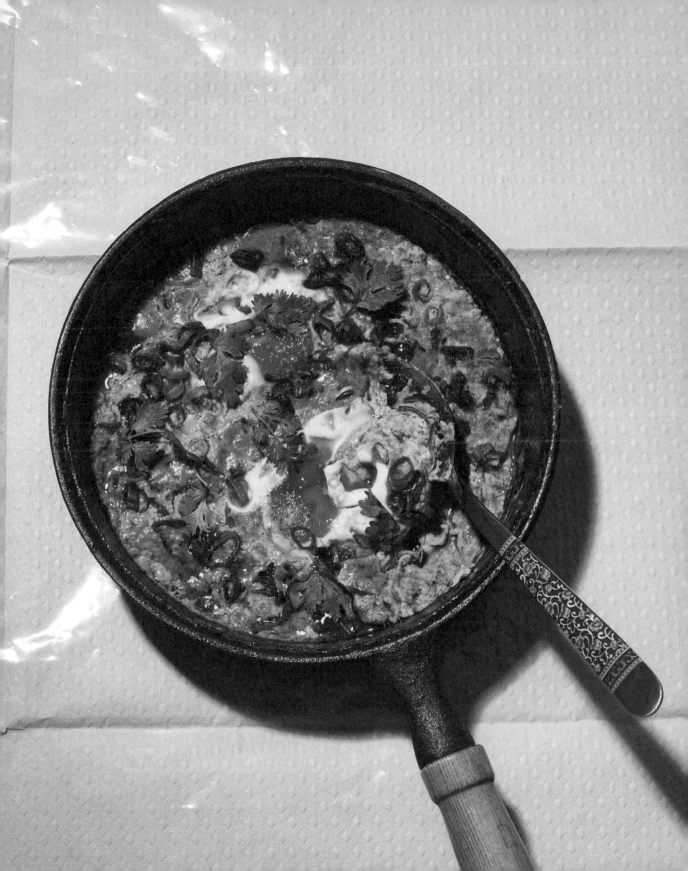

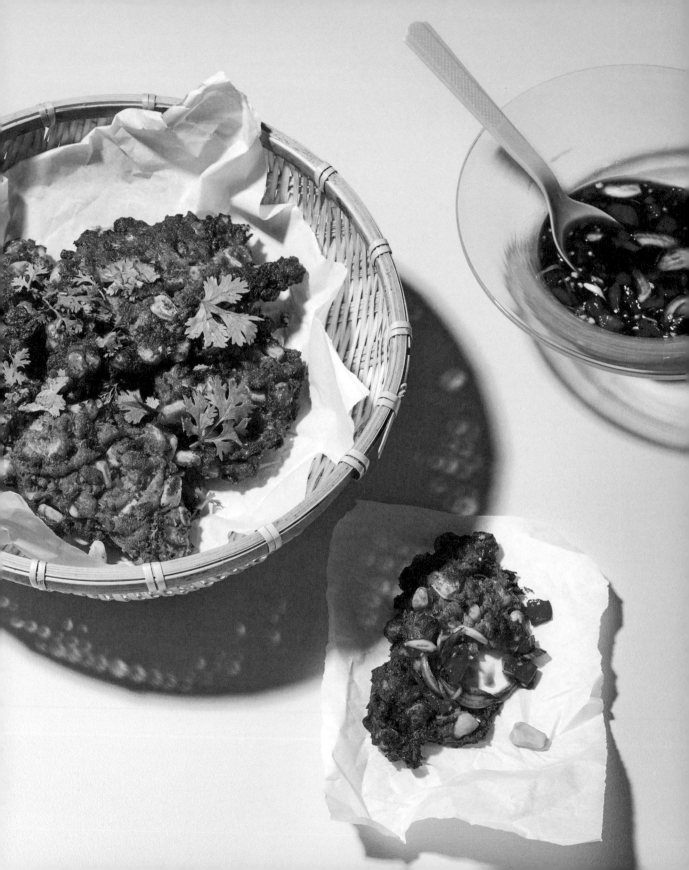

# TURMERIC CORN FRITTERS

## Ingredients

### Fritters

200 g (7 oz/1 cup) fresh corn kernels or tinned corn, drained

1 egg

2 garlic cloves

2 tsp ground turmeric or 2 cm (¾ in) piece of fresh turmeric

2 cm (¾ in) piece of fresh ginger root

1 tsp coriander seeds

1 tsp cumin seeds

1 tsp cayenne pepper

pinch of sea salt

2 spring onions (scallions), trimmed and chopped

½ celery stalk, grated

1 tbsp chopped coriander (cilantro)

1 small carrot, grated

20–30 g (¾–1 oz/scant ¼ cup) rice flour or cornflour

1 long red chilli, finely chopped

10 tbsp coconut oil, for deep-frying

### Dressing

4 tbsp kecap manis (Indonesian sweet soy sauce),

1 tbsp water

4 Thai chillies, thinly sliced

1 shallot, thinly sliced

**Serves 2**

**Vegetarian**

*Textured, spicy, moist and absolutely delicious, these fritters – also called **pedel jagung** – are great served with Ginger & Tomato Sambal (page 59) or kecap manis dressing diluted with a bit of water and sprinkled with chillies and shallots. Be good to yourself.*

## Method

Put half the corn kernels in a blender or food processor, along with the egg, garlic, turmeric, ginger, spices and a pinch of salt, and blitz until smooth.

Pour the mixture into a jug or bowl and add the rest of the fritter ingredients: the spring onions, celery, coriander, carrot, the remaining corn kernels, the rice flour or cornflour and chilli. Stir to combine.

Meanwhile, heat the coconut oil in a deep frying pan (skillet) over a medium-high heat until it reaches 160–180°C (320–350°F) (if it's any hotter, the fritters will burn before they are fully cooked through). If you don't have a thermometer, put a wooden spoon in the oil – as soon as bubbles start to come to the surface, the oil is ready. Add 1 heaped tablespoon per fritter to the hot oil, cooking in batches of four at a time, and fry for about 5 minutes on each side, turning them halfway, until golden brown. Remove with a slotted spoon and drain on paper towels and repeat with the rest of the batter.

Make the dressing by mixing all the ingredients together. Serve the warm fritters with the sauce.

# TURMERIC NASI GORENG

*Indonesian fried rice is typically eaten for breakfast. Packed with anti-inflammatory turmeric and ginger, this will put you right, quickly.*

## Method

Mix together the rice, kecap manis and tomato or hot sauce in a bowl. Set this aside.

Combine the spice paste ingredients (pounding them to a smoother consistency with a pestle and mortar if you prefer) in a bowl and set this aside.

Place a large wok or frying pan (skillet) over a medium–high heat and add the coconut oil. Once it has melted, add the spice paste to the pan, along with some salt and pepper. Stir-fry for 2–3 minutes until fragrant.

Add the rice to the pan, tossing and coating the rice with the spices until heated through. Feel free to add more kecap manis to taste.

Divide the rice between two bowls or plates and serve with the eggs (if using), cucumber, lime and sambal (if using).

## Ingredients

400 g (14 oz/generous 2 cups) cooked, cooled leftover rice

2 tbsp kecap manis (Indonesian sweet soy sauce), plus extra to taste

2 tbsp tomato passata, or hot sauce of any kind

2 tbsp coconut oil

sea salt and ground white pepper

## Spice Paste

2 shallots, finely chopped

2 cm (¾ in) piece of fresh turmeric, finely chopped

2 cm (¾ in) piece of fresh ginger root, finely chopped

1 garlic clove, finely chopped

2 red bird's eye chillies, finely chopped (optional)

## To Serve

2 eggs, soft-boiled (optional)

⅓ large cucumber, shredded or sliced, to serve

lime 'cheeks'

2 tbsp Ginger & Tomato Sambal (page 59), (optional)

**Serves 2**

**To make this vegetarian and vegan omit the anchovies from the sambal, adding extra salt if needed, and don't serve with the eggs**

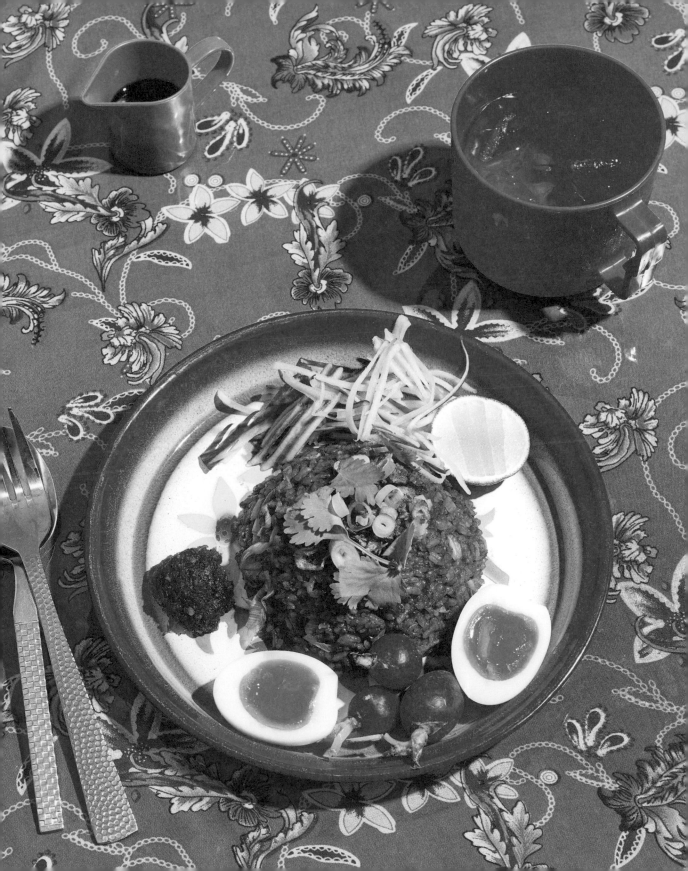

# GINGER & SESAME DAN DAN NOODLES

## Ingredients

500 g (1 lb 2 oz) spaghetti or medium egg noodles

500 ml (18 fl oz/2¼ cups) chicken stock or Cure-All Chicken Broth (page 144)

## Sauce

4 tbsp roasted sesame paste or peanut butter (smooth or crunchy)

4 tbsp soy sauce

4 tbsp rice vinegar

4 garlic cloves, finely chopped

2 tbsp honey

200–240 ml (7–8½ fl oz) Balancing Chilli Oil (page 49) or a store-bought chilli oil

## Pork

2 tbsp olive oil

450 g (1 lb) minced (ground) pork

2 tbsp finely chopped fresh ginger root

2 spring onions (scallions), white parts finely chopped, green parts sliced to serve

2 anchovy fillets (tinned in oil), finely chopped

2 tbsp Shaoxing wine or dry sherry

1 tsp unrefined cane sugar

## To Serve

50 g (2 oz) crushed peanuts

small bunch of coriander (cilantro), roughly chopped

Korean Turmeric Pickle (page 44) (optional), finely sliced

Serves 4

*This recipe reminds me of a Chinese-style spaghetti bolognese. And nothing beats spaghetti when it comes to times in need. The highly invigorating Balancing Chilli Oil (page 49) in the sauce is packed with ginger and citrussy Szechuan peppercorns that help to numb pain, boost your appetite, increase circulation and flush out toxins, as well as reduce inflammation. This recipe truly is a comforting and revitalising hug in a bowl.*

## Method

Whisk the first five sauce ingredients together in a bowl. Add the chilli oil to taste, then mix the sauce again. Set aside.

Cook the spaghetti or noodles in a pan of salted water according to the packet instructions. Drain and set aside.

Heat the oil in a wok or large non-stick frying pan (skillet) over a medium heat until hot. Add the pork and cook, breaking up the mince with a wooden spoon, until the meat has cooked through and any juices have evaporated. Turn down the heat, then add ginger, white part of the spring onion, anchovies, wine or sherry and sugar. Cook, stirring, for up to 20 minutes until all the liquid has evaporated and the pork turns a dark brown colour. Turn off the heat and set aside.

Bring the chicken stock to the boil in a saucepan. Once it reaches the boil, turn off the heat and set aside.

To serve, add 3 tablespoons of the sauce to each bowl, then share the pork between the four bowls. Divide the spaghetti or noodles into the bowls, then add a ladleful of warmed chicken stock to each bowl. Sprinkle each serving with peanuts, sliced green spring onion, coriander and pickle.

To eat, mix up the ingredients in each bowl until thoroughly combined. Add extra chilli oil if needed.

*Recipe photo overleaf*

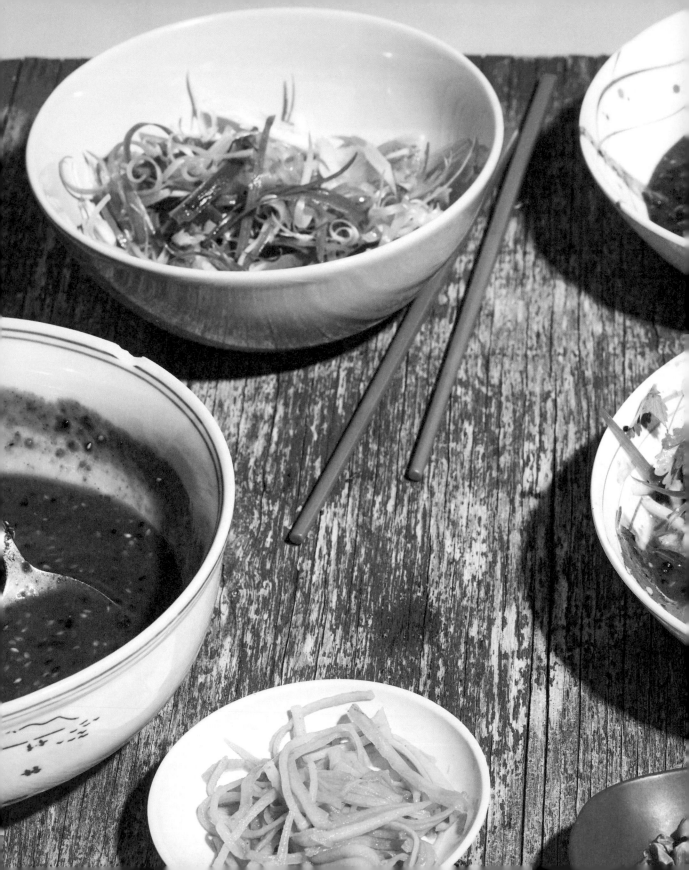

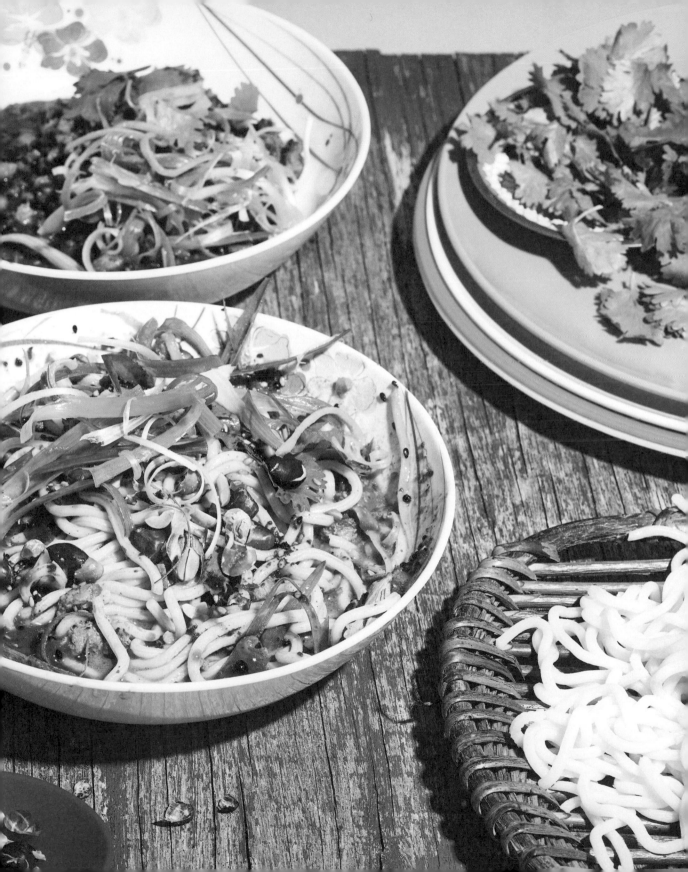

# KOREAN HANGOVER SOUP

〜〜〜〜〜〜〜〜〜〜〜

*Make a large batch of this soup before your next big night out; you'll be grateful you did. Koreans developed their own cure for heavy drinking centuries ago: a soup called* **haejang-guk**. *It literally means 'hangover soup'. The broth is rich and unquestionably beefy, but not over-the-top spicy, and aims to put you right, quickly. Enjoy with a warm bowl of rice and perhaps a Soy-Cured Egg Yolk (page 69), extra Gochujang (page 63) and Kimchi (page 52).*

## Method

Mix the soup base ingredients together in a small bowl.

Put the beef chuck or tofu in a separate bowl and add half of the soup base. Mix to coat and set aside for about 15 minutes.

Warm the broth in a saucepan over a low heat. Blanch the cabbage leaves in the broth for 1 minute, then remove with a slotted spoon and leave to cool before tearing the leaves into strips. Put the leaves in a bowl and add the rest of the soup base. Set aside.

Heat a large saucepan over a high heat. Add the marinated beef (or tofu) and radishes and cook for 1–2 minutes (you won't need any oil), then add the broth and the marinated cabbage. Stir and bring to the boil. Once it starts to boil, reduce the heat to medium and simmer for 20 minutes. (For the vegetarian option, just fry the radish for about a minute before adding the stock.)

Add the spring onions and bean sprouts, continue to simmer for 10 minutes, then remove from the heat, ladle into bowls and serve.

## Ingredients

750 g (1 lb 10 oz) beef chuck or firm tofu, sliced

1.5 litres (50 fl oz/6¼ cups) Veggie Healing Broth (page 146)

15 green cabbage leaves

200 g (7 oz) radishes, roughly chopped

2 spring onions (scallions), trimmed and cut into 4 cm (1½ in) pieces, plus shredded to garnish

3 handfuls of bean sprouts

## Soup Base

2 tbsp Gochujang (page 63)

6 garlic cloves, finely chopped

1 tbsp sesame oil

2 tbsp fish sauce (optional)

3 tbsp mirin

½ tsp ground black pepper

**Serves 2**

To make this vegetarian or vegan, substitute the beef chuck for tofu and omit the fish sauce, adding extra salt if needed

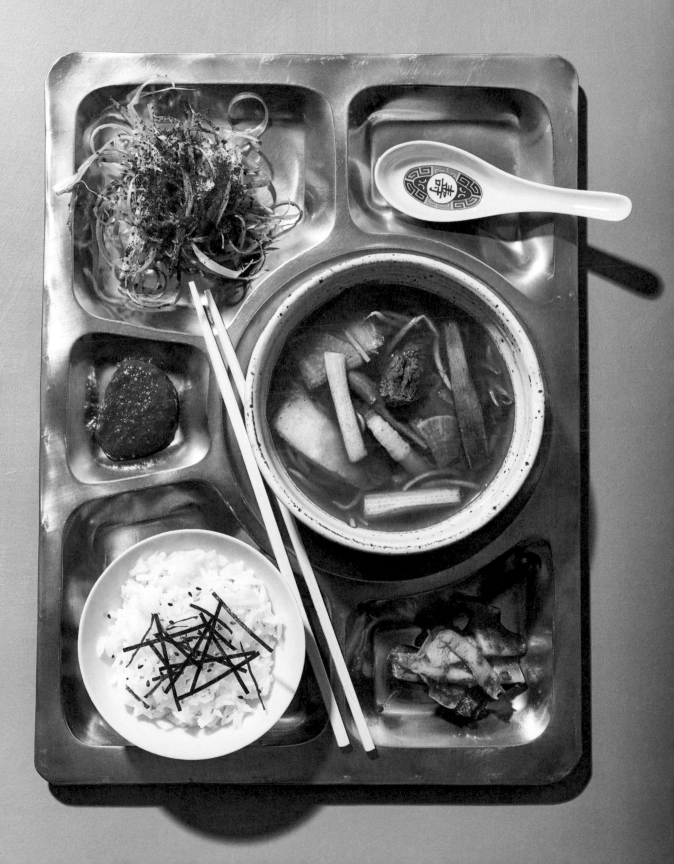

# BLOATED?

SOOTHE THE STOMACH WITH HUMBLE HERBS, SPICES & HOMEMADE PROBIOTICS. THESE RECIPES CONTAIN INGREDIENTS THAT HAVE POTENT DIGESTIVE BENEFITS & HAVE BEEN USED TO ALLEVIATE GAS, BLOATING & STOMACH PAINS FOR CENTURIES. THEY NATURALLY STIMULATE THE BODY'S DIGESTIVE ENZYMES & HELP TO RELIEVE INFLAMMATION & DISCOMFORT.

# THAI PAPAYA SALAD

## Ingredients

⅓ small (cannonball) green cabbage, thinly sliced

handful of green beans, trimmed and halved

handful of coriander (cilantro), chopped

100 g (3½ oz/scant ⅔ cup) roasted peanuts, crushed

## Dressing

2 cm (¾ in) piece of fresh ginger root

½ garlic clove

2 small red Thai chillies

5 cherry tomatoes

2 tbsp fish sauce (optional)

juice of 1 lime

2 tbsp coconut sugar

**Som tam** *or Thai papaya salad is well known for being simultaneously salty, sweet, spicy, sour and bitter. Papaya salad is certainly one of my favourite street food snacks. Green papaya is hard to come by, however, so I use hard green cabbage instead. This salad is addictively fiery – go easy on the chilli if you like.*

## Method

First make the dressing by smashing the dressing ingredients together with a medium-large pestle and mortar: start with the ginger, garlic and chillies. Add the cherry tomatoes and lightly squash them, then mix in the liquids and sugar. Taste as you go – you're looking for a balanced flavour. You may want to adjust the ingredient quantities to your liking.

Once you are happy, add the cabbage to the mortar bit by bit, bashing it lightly into the sauce. Add the green beans and lightly bash those too, then add the coriander and crushed peanuts. Serve straight away.

### Serves 2

**To make this vegetarian and vegan, omit the fish sauce from the dressing, adding extra salt if needed**

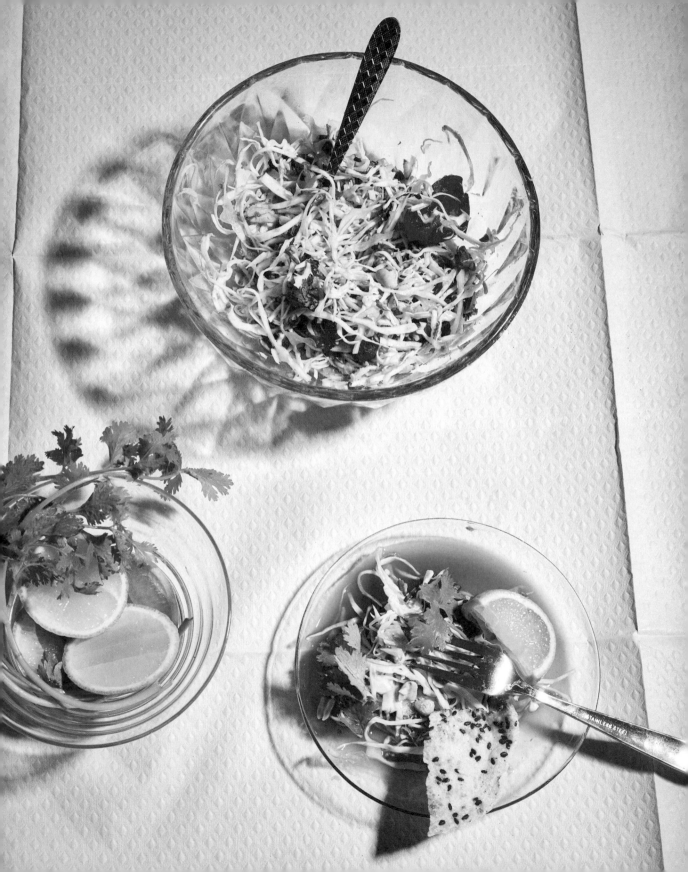

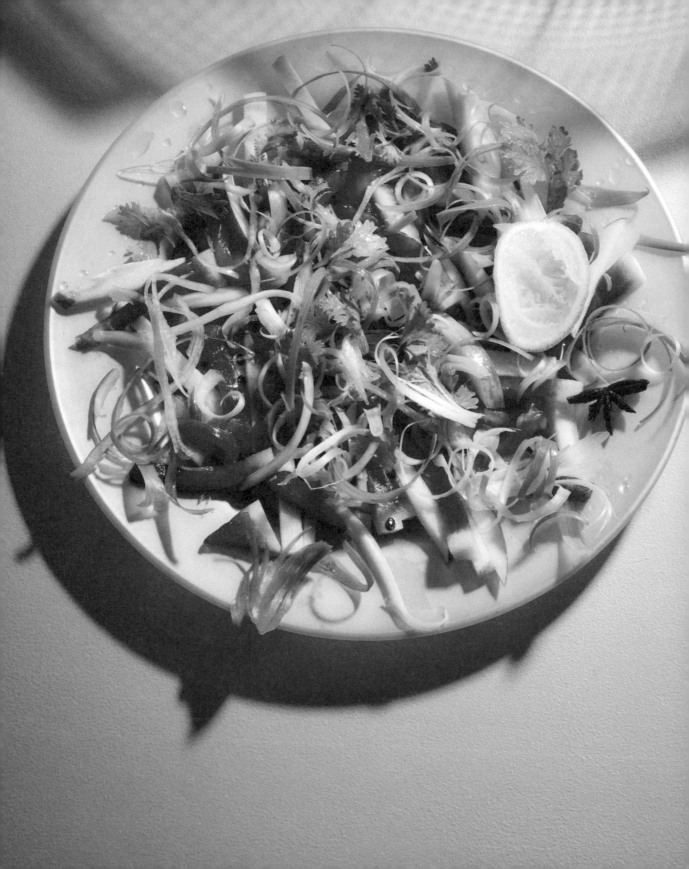

# SPICY PICKLED WATERMELON SALAD

### Ingredients

1.5 kg (3 lb 5 oz) rindless watermelon, sliced

1 green apple, cut into thin slices

1 fresh jalapeño, thinly sliced (optional)

1 spring onion (scallion), trimmed and thinly sliced

bunch of coriander (cilantro), chopped

juice of 1 lime

### Brine

200 g (7 oz/generous 1 cup) unrefined cane sugar

200 ml (7 fl oz/scant 1 cup) apple cider vinegar

1 long red or green chilli, finely chopped

25 g (¾ oz) fresh ginger root, sliced

2 whole star anise

1 tbsp sea salt

1 tsp black peppercorns

1 tsp fennel seeds

1 bay leaf

1 lime, quartered

200 ml (7 fl oz/scant 1 cup) water

Serves 2

Vegetarian

Vegan

*This dish contains a perfect balance of cooling and warming ingredients. Packed with pickled, tangy, fruity and spicy flavours, it's perfect in the summer. Start making the brine the day before you plan to tuck in.*

### Method

Start by making the brine: put all the ingredients in a medium saucepan. Bring to the boil over a medium heat, stirring until the sugar dissolves. As soon as it reaches boiling point, turn off the heat. Allow the brine to cool.

Put the watermelon into a clean 1 litre (34 fl oz/ 4 cup) container or jar and fill it with the cooled brine. The brine needs to cover the watermelon, so take some pieces out if necessary. Seal and leave the watermelon to pickle in the fridge overnight.

The next day, remove all the watermelon from the brine and slice into bite-sized chunks.

Gently toss the watermelon, apple, jalapeño (if using), spring onion, coriander and lime juice in a large bowl and serve.

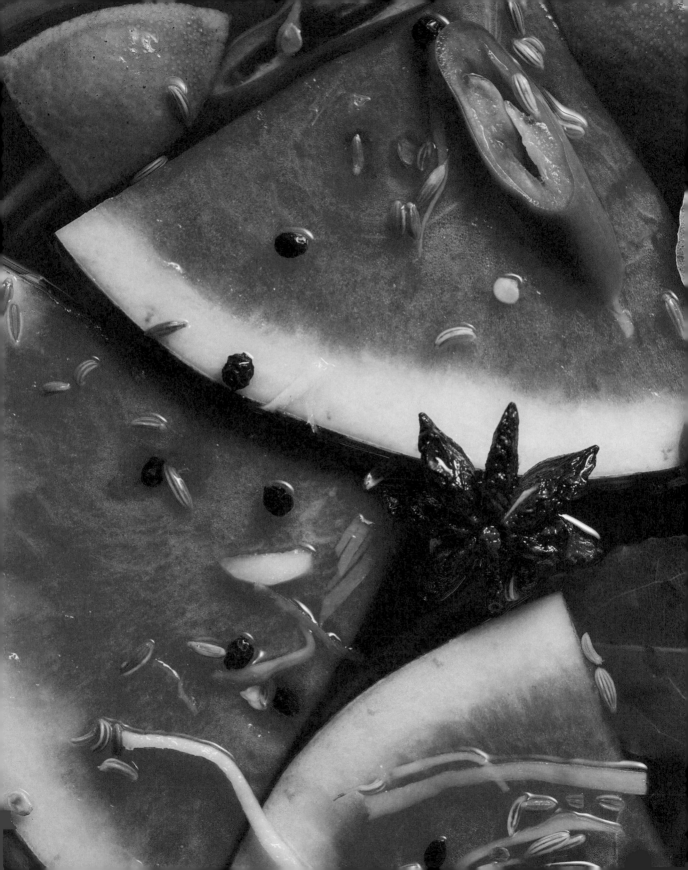

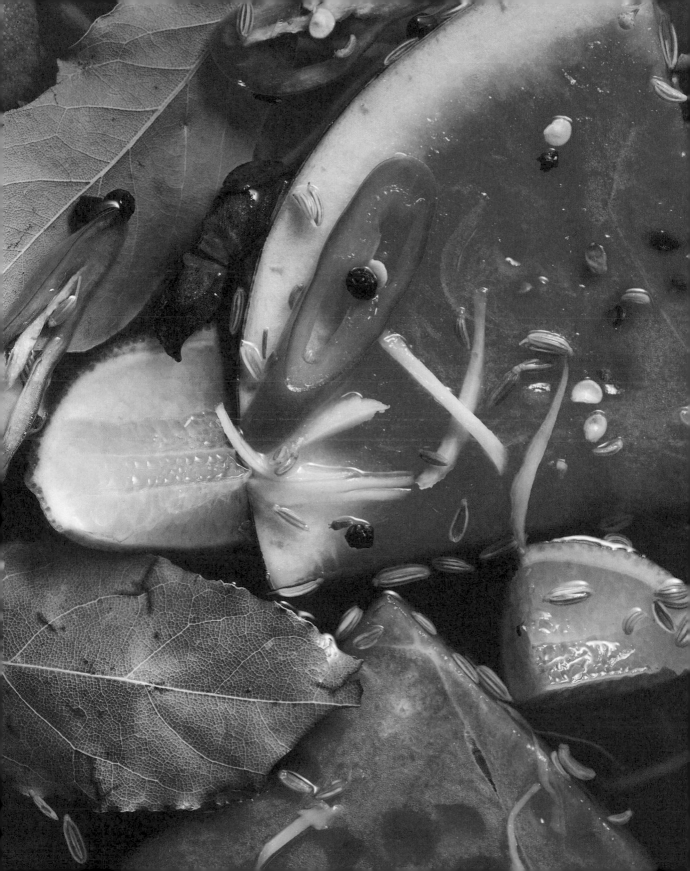

# GINGER & BLACK PEPPER SALMON

*This dish shares similarities with Singapore black pepper crab. Black pepper and ginger are considered very important healing spices in Ayurveda. Together, they're known as **trikatu**; a blend of spices that work in synergy to stimulate the digestive fire. I serve this with steamed rice.*

## Method

Heat the oil in a large frying pan (skillet) over a medium-high heat, add the salmon and fry (in batches if necessary – don't overcrowd the pan), turning the pieces until they are golden all over, then transfer to a plate to rest.

Wipe the pan to remove any traces of salmon or oil and throw in the butter. Once it has melted, add the shallots, chillies, garlic and ginger. Fry over a low-medium heat, stirring occasionally, for up to 15 minutes, making sure they don't colour, until everything looks shiny and is completely soft.

Add the kecap manis, soy sauce and sugar to the pan of softened shallots, stir, then add the crushed pepper. Add the salmon to the pan to warm it through for about a minute, then stir in the spring onions. Serve immediately with cooked rice and shredded spring onions.

## Ingredients

glug of olive oil

2 skinless salmon fillets, cut into bite-sized squares

70 g (2½ oz) unsalted butter

125 g (4 oz) small shallots (about 5), thinly sliced

2 large red chillies, thinly sliced

5 garlic cloves, finely chopped

1½ tbsp finely chopped fresh ginger root

1½ tbsp kecap manis (Indonesian sweet soy sauce)

3 tbsp soy sauce

1 tbsp unrefined cane sugar

1½–2 tbsp coarsely ground black peppercorns

6 spring onions (scallions), trimmed and cut into 3 cm- (1¼ in-) long pieces, plus shredded to serve

cooked rice, to serve

**Serves 2**

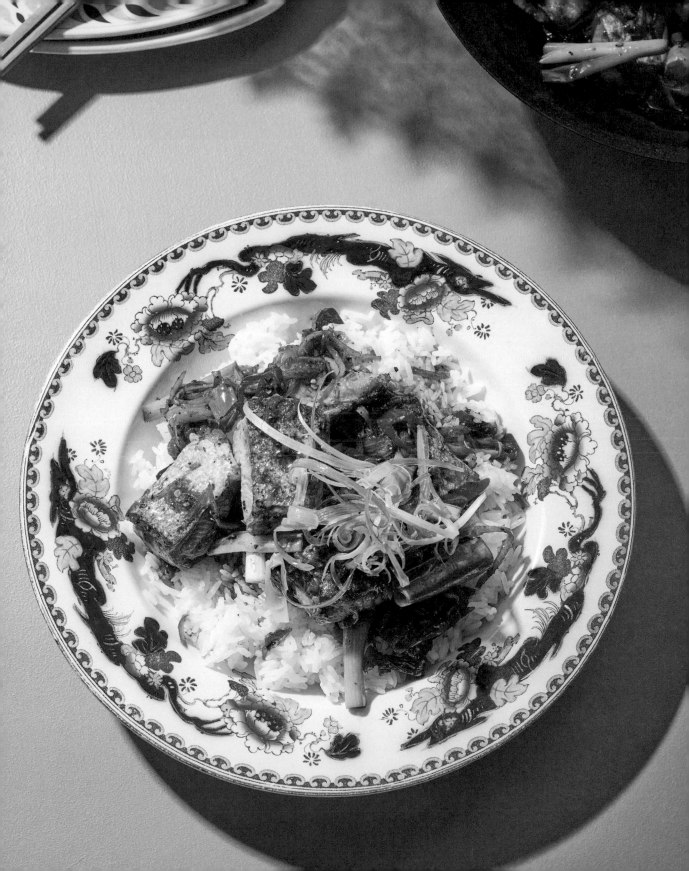

# BIBIMBAP WRAPS

### Ingredients

150 g (5 oz) good-quality minced (ground) beef or mushrooms, thickly sliced

½ carrot, courgette (zucchini) or cucumber (or a combination of all three), julienned

pinch of sea salt

2 tbsp coconut oil

Gochujang (page 63) or Kimchi Miso Sauce (page 56)

perilla leaves or lettuce cups

2 portions of cooled, cooked rice

1 spring onion (scallion), shredded

100 g (3½ oz) bean sprouts

### Marinade

1 tbsp crushed or finely chopped garlic

3 tbsp soy sauce

1½ tbsp honey

½ tsp freshly ground black pepper

1 tsp sesame seeds

2 tsp sesame oil

### Dressing

1 tsp crushed garlic

2 tsp sesame oil

1 tsp sesame seeds

pinch of sea salt

**Serves 2**

To make ths vegetarian, use the mushrooms instead of beef and omit the kimchi miso sauce

*Bibimbap derives from* **goldongban** *(a bowl of rice mixed with vegetables, meat and sauce), which dates back to some time between the 14th and 16th centuries.*

*Traditionally, it was eaten on the eve of the lunar new year, when people would clear out their pantries, using up whatever was left over by chucking it into their rice bowls, tossing it together, and calling it dinner. The idea that you can consciously create a dish with such a rich history just by throwing all your leftovers into a bowl of rice really makes me happy.*

*I like to serve my bibimbap in perilla leaves (but lettuce cups work great too) and dunk it straight into the Gochujang (page 63), or Kimchi Miso Sauce (page 56). Double dipping's your call. As is the type of 'wrap' you want to use. Adapt the vegetables to suit what you have in your fridge and the season.*

## Method

Combine the marinade ingredients in a bowl. Add the beef or mushrooms and leave to marinate for at least 30 minutes while you are doing the rest of your prep.

Put the julienned carrot, courgette or cucumber in a bowl and mix with a pinch of salt. Leave to stand at room temperature for 5–10 minutes until they start to 'sweat', then rinse under cold running water and squeeze to remove the water.

Combine the dressing ingredients in a bowl, add the julienned vegetable(s) and mix with your hands. Keep all of the veggies separate or combine them together for ease. Set aside.

Melt the coconut oil in a frying pan (skillet) over a medium heat, add the marinated beef or mushrooms and fry for about 10 minutes until all the marinade has been absorbed and the beef or mushrooms are cooked through and golden.

Add some water to the gochujang paste or kimchi miso sauce until it reaches your desired consistency.

Now you're ready to eat. Grab a perilla leaf or lettuce cup, smear it with gochujang paste or kimchi miso sauce, top with a bit of cooked rice, the beef or mushrooms, the dressed vegetables, spring onions and bean sprouts.

*Recipe photo overleaf*

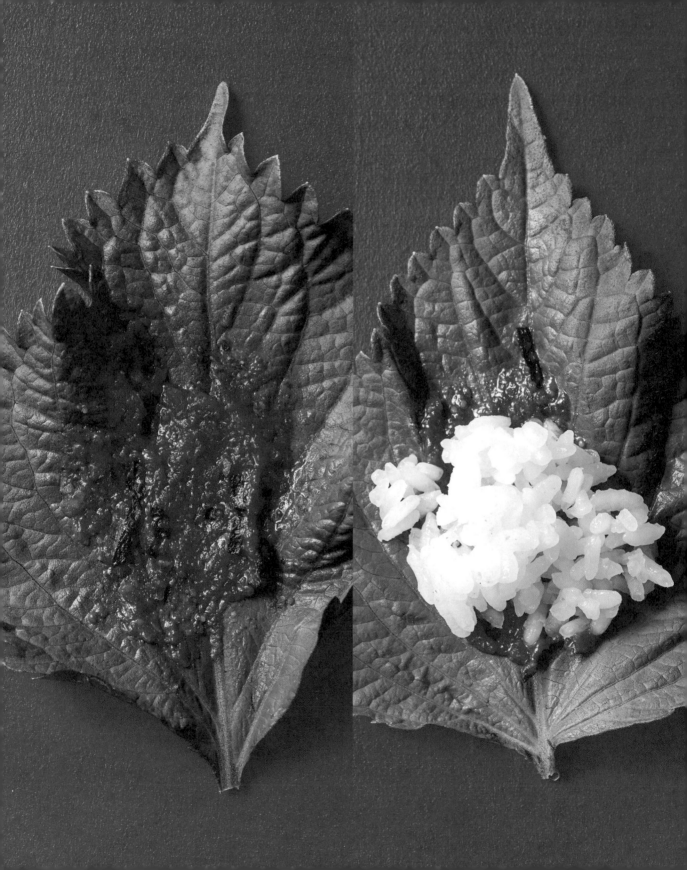

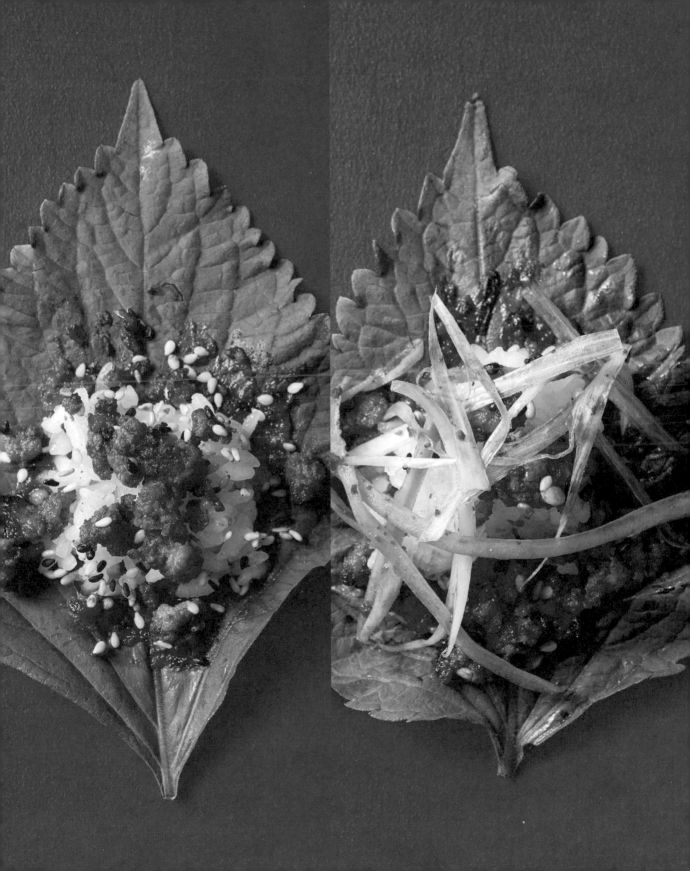

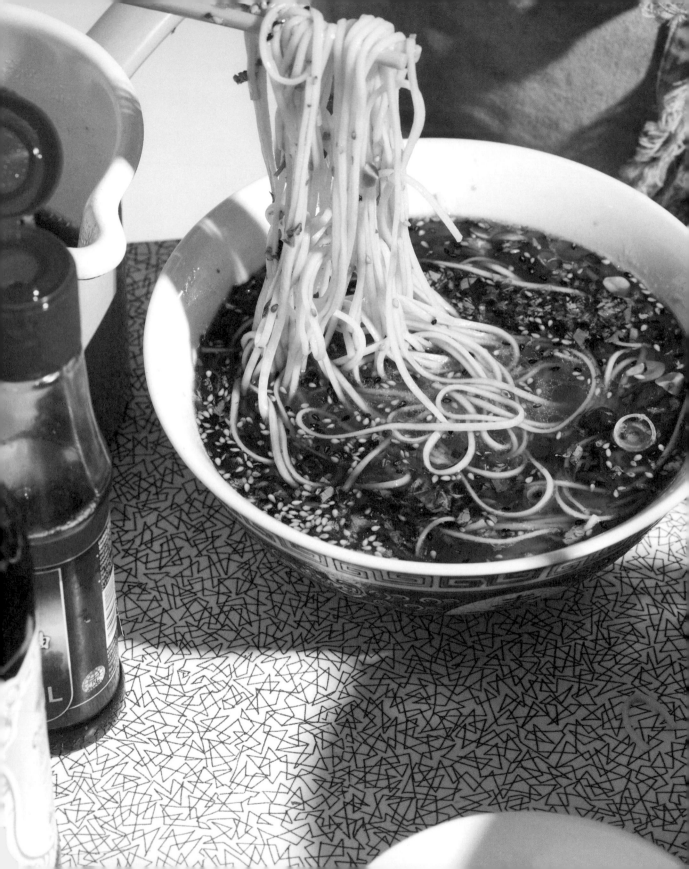

# NUMBINGLY SOOTHING NOODLES

### Ingredients

½ tsp black rice vinegar

2 tbsp soy sauce

1 spring onion (scallion), white part finely chopped, green part roughly chopped

2 small garlic cloves, finely chopped

2 tsp finely chopped fresh ginger root

4 tbsp Balancing Chilli Oil (page 49)

2 tsp sesame oil

4 tsp lard or coconut oil

pinch of sea salt

300 g (10½ oz) thin dried egg noodles

500 ml (18 fl oz/2¼ cups) Veggie Healing Broth (pages 146) or Cure-All Chicken Broth (page 144) or water

2 tbsp smashed roasted peanuts

2 tbsp chopped coriander (cilantro)

**Serves 2**

**To make this vegetarian, substitute the lard for coconut oil and use veggie broth**

*The rounded flavour of the zingy Szechuan peppercorns in this mouth- and stomach-numbing Xiomian-style noodle soup will make you feel as though you're carrying a hot-water bottle in your stomach – in a good way.*

### Method

Divide the vinegar, soy sauce, finely chopped white part of the spring onion, garlic, ginger, chilli oil, sesame oil, lard (or coconut oil) and a pinch of salt between two serving bowls.

Cook the noodles in boiling water according to the packet instructions, then drain and divide them between the two serving bowls. Heat the stock or water, then pour enough into the serving bowls to cover the noodles.

Garnish each serving with the peanuts, green part of the spring onion and chopped coriander. Add more chilli oil if you like it hotter!

# PROBIOTIC KIMCHI FRIED GRAINS

**Kimchi bokkeumbap** *(Korean fried rice) is ridiculously easy to make, delicious and packed with gut-healing ingredients like probiotic kimchi and ginger. You can use any leftover grains, such as rice, barley and quinoa. I like a 50/50 combination of rice and barley.*

## Method

Sauté the lardons (if using) in the coconut oil or butter in a large wok or frying pan (skillet) over a medium-high heat, just before they become crispy (if you're not using lardons simply heat the oil or butter). Add the onion, garlic and ginger, then sauté over a medium heat for about 5 minutes, until they become aromatic and the lardons are crisp.

Add the chopped kimchi, grains and gochujang, and cook, stirring frequently, for about 5 minutes, until everything is mixed through evenly and is piping hot.

Reduce the heat to medium-low, flatten the rice in the pan with a spatula and cook for a further 2 minutes. The bottom of the rice will take on a nice crispy consistency. The longer you leave it, the more crispy the bottom will become.

Serve the rice with a fried or soy-cured egg yolks, sprinkled with the sliced spring onion.

## Ingredients

100 g (3½ oz) smoked bacon lardons (optional)

1 tbsp coconut oil or butter

1 small onion, finely chopped

2 garlic cloves, finely chopped

2 cm (¾ in) piece of fresh ginger root, finely chopped

150 g (5 oz) Easy Probiotic Kimchi (page 52), chopped

300 g (10½ oz) cooked grains of choice, preferably a day old

1 tbsp Gochujang (page 63)

## To Serve

2 eggs, fried or Soy-Cured Egg Yolks (page 69)

2 spring onions (scallions), trimmed and thinly sliced

Serves 2

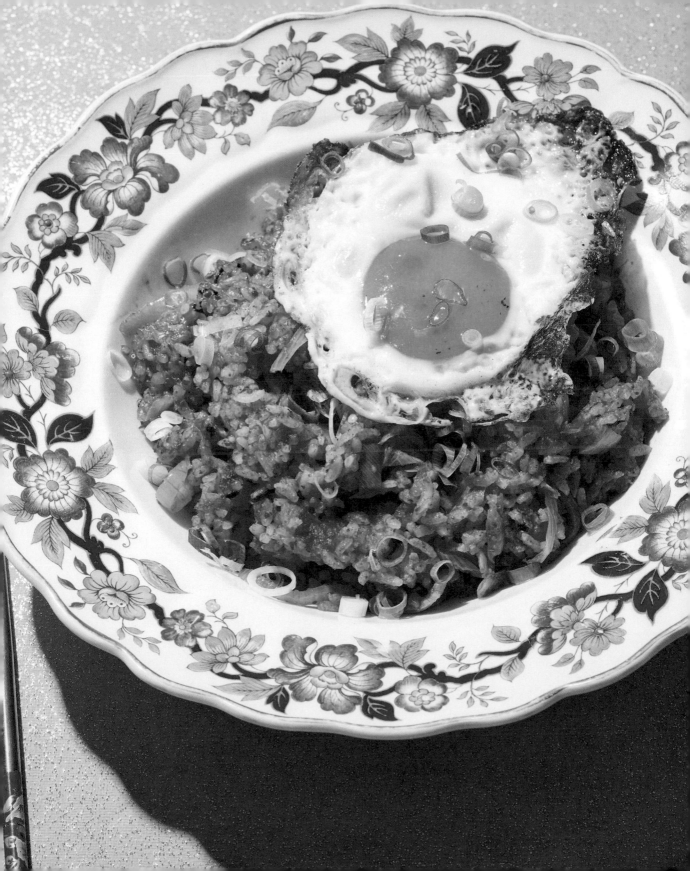

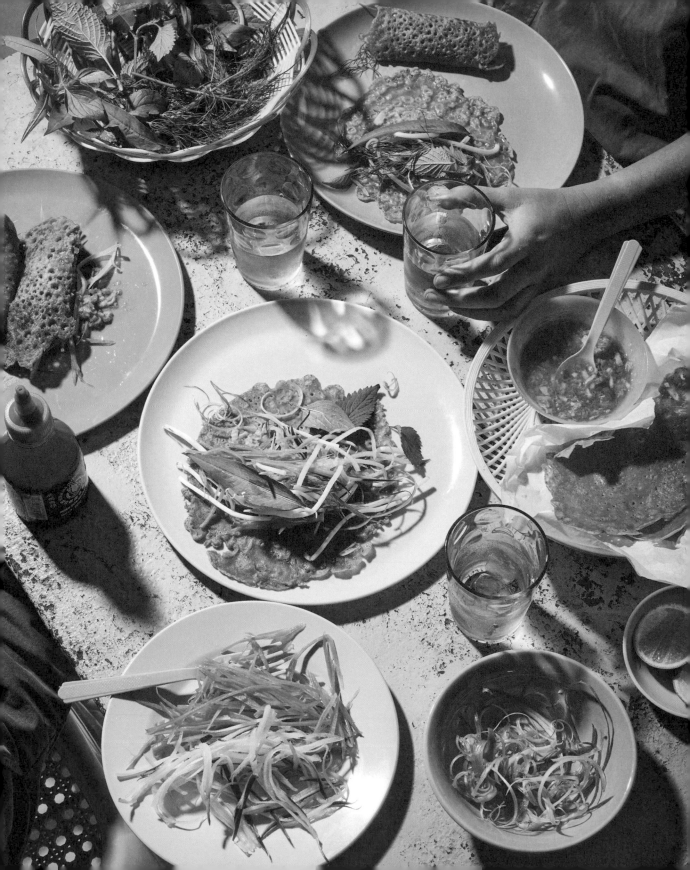

# HERB & TURMERIC PANCAKES

## Ingredients

### Pancake Batter (makes 15)

200 g (7 oz/generous 1 cup) rice flour

240 ml (8½ fl oz/1 cup) full-fat coconut milk

240 ml (8½ fl oz/1 cup) cold water

pinch of unrefined sugar

½ tsp sea salt

2 tsp ground turmeric

2 tbsp coconut oil, for frying

### Filling

2 carrots, julienned

1 cucumber, julienned

2 spring onions (scallions), trimmed and thinly sliced

small bunch each of mint, coriander (cilantro) and Thai basil

### Sauce

juice of 2 limes

1 tsp sesame oil

1 tbsp coconut sugar

2 tsp grated fresh ginger root

1 red chilli, finely chopped

1 garlic clove, crushed

½ tsp sea salt

### To Serve

lime wedges

Probiotic Sriracha (page 65) or store-bought (optional)

Serves 5

Vegetarian

Vegan

*I discovered these sizzling anti-inflammatory turmeric pancakes – also called **banh xeo** – from Vietnam, packed with the freshest aromatic herbs and a zingy dipping sauce, at Kylie Kwong's stall at Carriageworks Farmers Market in Sydney, Australia, and never looked back.*

## Method

Start by making the pancake batter: mix all the batter ingredients together, except for the oil, in a large bowl. The batter should be runny like crêpe batter. Heat a non-stick frying pan (skillet) over a medium heat, lightly grease with some of the coconut oil, then pour in a ladle of batter and swirl to coat the base of the pan (the pancakes should be very thin). Cook the pancake until tiny holes start to appear on the surface and it colours lightly on the underside, then flip and cook on the other side until coloured on both sides. Repeat with the rest of the batter, and extra coconut oil as necessary. Once you've cooked them all, let them cool and keep to one side.

Combine the filling ingredients in a bowl. Then, in a separate bowl, whisk the sauce ingredients together. Add the sauce to the filling and toss to combine.

To serve, fill the cooled pancakes with the dressed filling, roll up and serve alongside wedges of lime and maybe some sriracha too.

# DIGESTIVE HERB SALAD

*Herbs like dill, coriander and mint, and spices like ginger, have been used in traditional systems of medicine to aid digestion for thousands of years. They are gentle yet powerful. Inspired by Thailand, this herb salad helps beat the bloat and reboot the natural strength of the digestive system. Kill two birds with one stone – eat your medicine, heal through food.*

## Method

Mix the coconut oil, lime juice, ginger, fish sauce (if using), red chilli, white pepper and sugar together in a bowl. Then add the herbs and avocado (if using), and mix together using your hands, then serve.

## Ingredients

1 tbsp coconut oil, melted

juice of 1 lime

2 cm (¾ in) piece of fresh ginger root, finely chopped

2 tsp fish sauce (optional)

1 small red Thai chilli, finely diced

pinch of ground white pepper

¼ tsp palm sugar or unrefined cane sugar

handful of mint, leaves only

handful of dill, roughly chopped

handful of coriander (cilantro), roughly chopped

handful of Thai basil, leaves only

½ ripe avocado, chopped (optional)

**Serves 2**

**To make this vegetarian or vegan, omit the fish sauce, adding extra salt if needed**

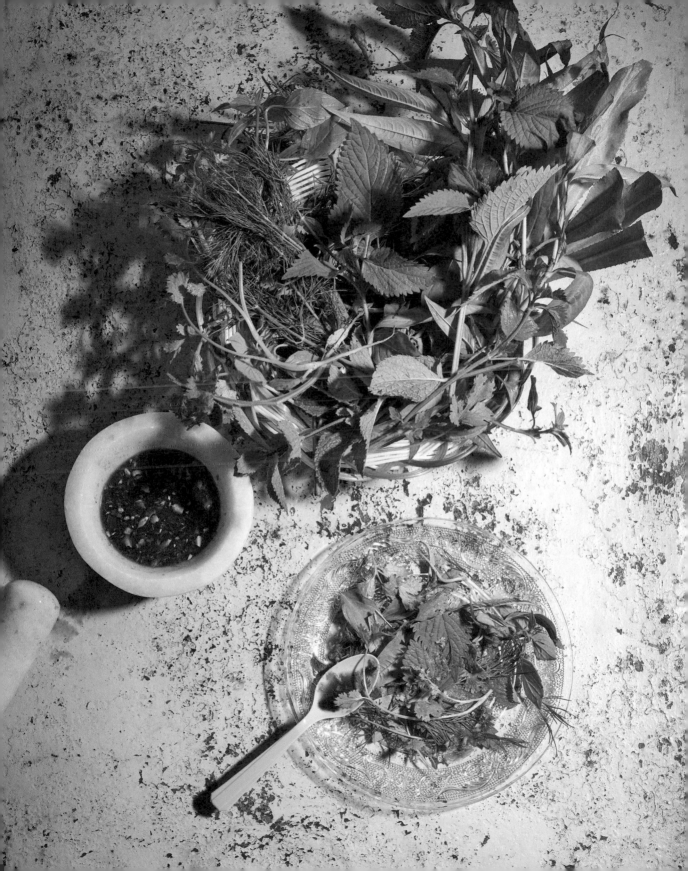

# SICK?

HERE'S EVERYTHING YOU NEED TO
GET YOU THROUGH FLU SEASON.
AS THE CHILL SETS IN, RATHER THAN
REACH FOR THE FLU TABLETS, PULL OUT
THE INGREDIENTS FOR JAMU NOODLE SOUP,
THE ORIGINAL COLD CURE & NATURAL
IMMUNE BOOSTER. ALL OF THESE RECIPES
ARE AS COMFORTING AS THEY ARE
HEALING, & PACKED WITH POTENT ANTI-
INFLAMMATORY INGREDIENTS & FLAVOUR.

# RESTORATIVE CONGEE

## THE ULTIMATE COMFORT FOOD

*This is a dish for that time you need to eat your feelings. Congee is a traditional Chinese healing porridge. It's easy on the digestive system, packed with energy and forms the ideal base for a number of therapeutic foods you can pile on top. It's the perfect recovery recipe that will warm the body, nourish and soothe the digestive system, rehydrate and give you strength. I prefer making this with black rice but feel free to use any variety you like.*

## Method

Put the rice and broth or water in a saucepan, add a pinch of salt, bring to the boil, then cook at a low simmer for 1–1½ hours until the rice is creamy but still a bit loose. If it thickens too much, add more stock or water. Adjust the seasoning to taste with salt, soy sauce and a dash of rice wine vinegar.

Meanwhile, heat the coconut oil in a large frying pan (skillet) over a medium-high heat. Add the garlic and ginger and cook until the edges start to turn golden, then add the mushrooms and a pinch of salt and cook until golden (try not to stir them too much). Stir in the spinach, turn off the heat, cover, let the spinach wilt, then remove the lid again.

To serve, divide the congee among four bowls and dust it with white pepper. Top with the fried mushrooms and spinach, sprinkle with the herbs, and an extra splash of soy sauce too.

The addition of a soft-boiled egg, pickles and chilli oil brings it all together perfectly.

## Ingredients

180 g (6 oz/generous ¾ cup) black rice, washed

1.5 litres (50 fl oz/6 ¼ cups) Cure-All Chicken Broth (page 144), Veggie Healing Broth (page 146) or water

2 tbsp soy sauce, or to taste

2 tbsp rice wine vinegar, or to taste

2 tsp coconut oil

1 large garlic clove, finely chopped

2 cm (¾ in) piece of fresh ginger root, peeled and finely chopped

handful of shiitake mushrooms, sliced

handful of spinach, roughly chopped

sea salt and freshly ground white pepper

## To Serve

handful of roughly torn or chopped mint and coriander (cilantro) (I like a 50/50 mix)

soft-boiled egg, peeled, doused with soy sauce and halved (optional)

pickles (optional)

Balancing Chilli Oil (page 49)

**Serves 4**

**To make this vegetarian, substitute the chicken broth with veggie broth or water**

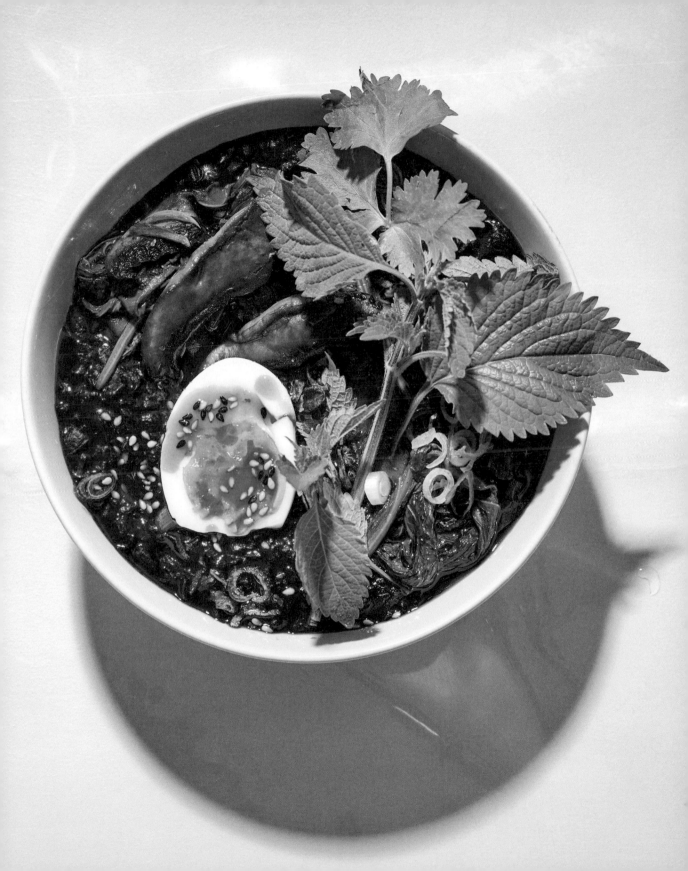

# IMMUNITY-BOOSTING TURMERIC DHAL

## Ingredients

### Turmeric Dhal

300 g (10½ oz/1⅓ cups) chana dhal (split peas), rinsed

3 tbsp coconut oil or ghee

1 onion, finely chopped

2 garlic cloves, finely grated

5 cm (2 in) piece of fresh ginger root, peeled and finely grated

½ tsp ground cardamom

2 tsp ground coriander

1 tsp chilli powder

3 cm (1¼ in) piece of fresh turmeric, finely grated, or 2 tsp ground turmeric

6 tbsp tomato purée

1.25 litres (42 fl oz/generous 5 cups) cold water

### Lime-Pickled Onion

1 lime

1 small red onion, very thinly sliced into rounds and rinsed

1 tsp unrefined cane sugar

### Salted Coconut Yoghurt

150 g (5 oz/generous ½ cup) coconut yoghurt or plain cow's milk yoghurt (optional)

2 tbsp cold water

generous pinch of sea salt

### To Serve

250 g (9 oz/1¼ cup) rice of choice, cooked

handful of coriander (cilantro), chopped

Serves 4

To make this vegan, use coconut yoghurt or omit completely

*Traditional wisdom about food and its therapeutic effects has been established for many generations in India. Dhal is India's favourite comfort food and the cornerstone to any Ayurvedic diet. It's satisfying and nourishing, yet light. The spices stimulate your appetite and digestive fire, as well as restore your energy levels and give your immune system a boost.*

## Method

Soak the chana dhal in a deep bowl of cold water for at least a few hours (ideally overnight).

When you're ready to cook, prepare the pickled onion. Finely zest the lime into a small bowl, then halve the lime and squeeze in the juice. Add the onion slices and sugar, then stir to combine. Leave this at room temperature until ready to serve.

To cook the dhal, add the coconut oil or ghee to a large saucepan over a medium heat, add the chopped onion and fry gently for 10–15 minutes, until sweet, soft and lightly browned. Add the garlic, ginger, cardamom, ground coriander, chilli powder, turmeric and tomato purée and stir for a couple of minutes.

Drain the chana dhal and add them to the pan with the cold water. Bring to the boil, then turn the heat down to a fairly gentle simmer, put the lid on and cook for 1½ hours, or longer if needed, until the dhal is thick and deeply flavoured, stirring from time to time. Top it up with a little hot water from the kettle if it looks too dry.

Mix the yoghurt and water in a small bowl, and season with salt.

Serve the dhal, yoghurt and lime-pickled onion with fluffy rice and some fresh coriander.

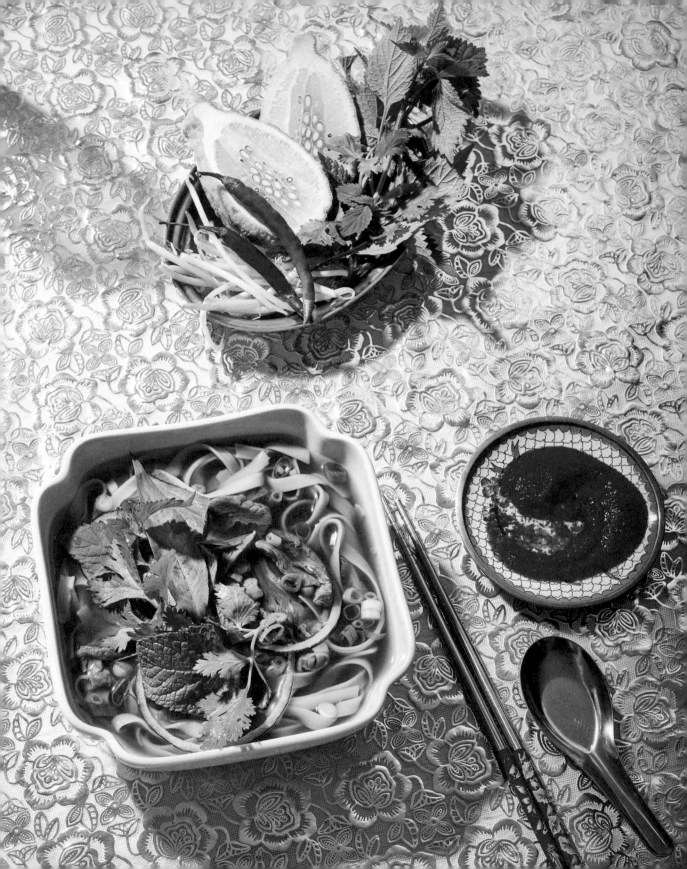

# CURE-ALL BEEF PHO

〰〰〰〰〰〰〰〰〰

## Ingredients

1 large onion (skin on)

6 cm (2½ in) piece of fresh ginger root (skin on)

3.5 litres (120 fl oz/15 cups) beef stock

1 tbsp coconut sugar or unrefined cane sugar

pinch of ground white pepper

6 cm (2½ in) piece of Vietnamese or regular cinnamon

1 star anise

1 clove

1 black cardamom pod (optional)

3 tbsp fish sauce, or to taste

sea salt

400 g (14 oz) flank steak, sliced thinly against the grain

### Turmeric Rice Noodles

200 g (7 oz) flat, dry rice noodles

1 tbsp ground turmeric

### To Serve

6 spring onions (scallions), trimmed and thinly sliced

small bunch of coriander (cilantro), chopped

Thai basil leaves

red onion, thinly sliced

limes, sliced

Probiotic Sriracha (optional) (page 65)

**Serves 4**

*This miraculous bowl of soup from Vietnam can cure almost anything. Nothing is more comforting than a bowl of pho, especially when you're feeling under the weather. Pho is a typical Vietnamese breakfast, perfect for jump-starting your immune system or lifting your spirits on a dreary day. Vietnamese food is known to be one of the healthiest in the world because of the importance placed on balance (through yin and yang) to create food that is nutritious and delicious at the same time. The flank steak needs to be sliced paper thin as it is served raw – it is cooked by the heat of the piping hot broth.*

## Method

Preheat the oven to 180°C (350°F/gas 4).

Put the onion and ginger in a roasting tray (pan) and roast for about 1 hour until soft to the touch. Remove from the oven and allow to cool, then peel the onion, cut it in half and slice the ginger.

Add the beef stock to a large saucepan or stockpot, along with the roasted onion and ginger, sugar, white pepper, cinnamon, star anise, clove and black cardamom pod (if using). Bring to the boil, then reduce the heat and simmer for 30–40 minutes.

Strain the broth, then return it to the pan and bring back to the boil. Season with fish sauce and salt, to taste.

Soak the rice noodles in a bowl of hot water until soft (or according to the packet instructions), then drain.

Bring a saucepan of water to the boil, add the rice noodles and cook for 3–4 minutes, then add the turmeric and stir. Drain again and rinse under cold running water until cool. Drain well.

Divide the noodles evenly among four warmed bowls. Pour two ladles of broth over the noodles and top with the thinly cut steak and garnishes.

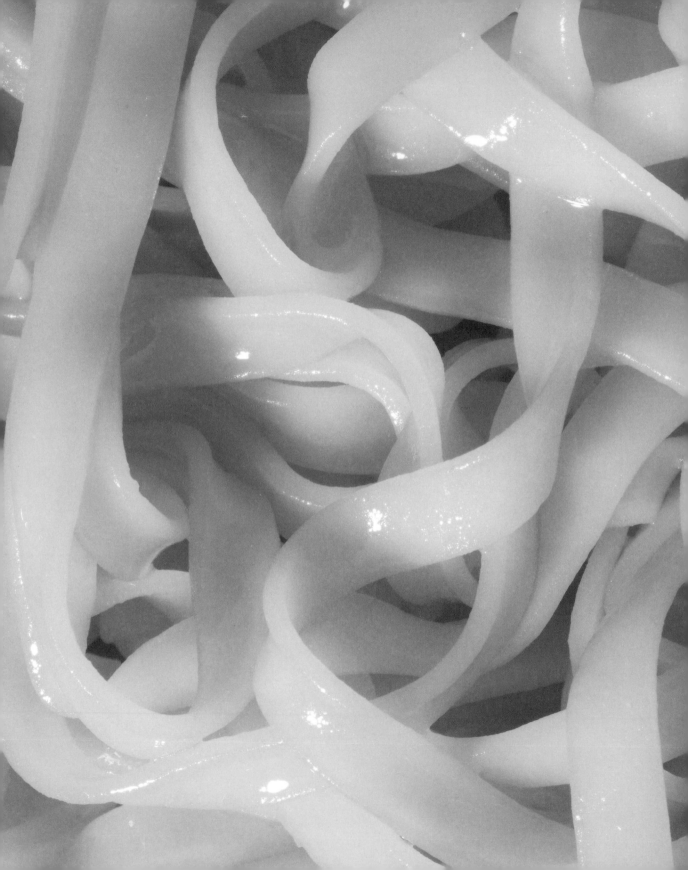

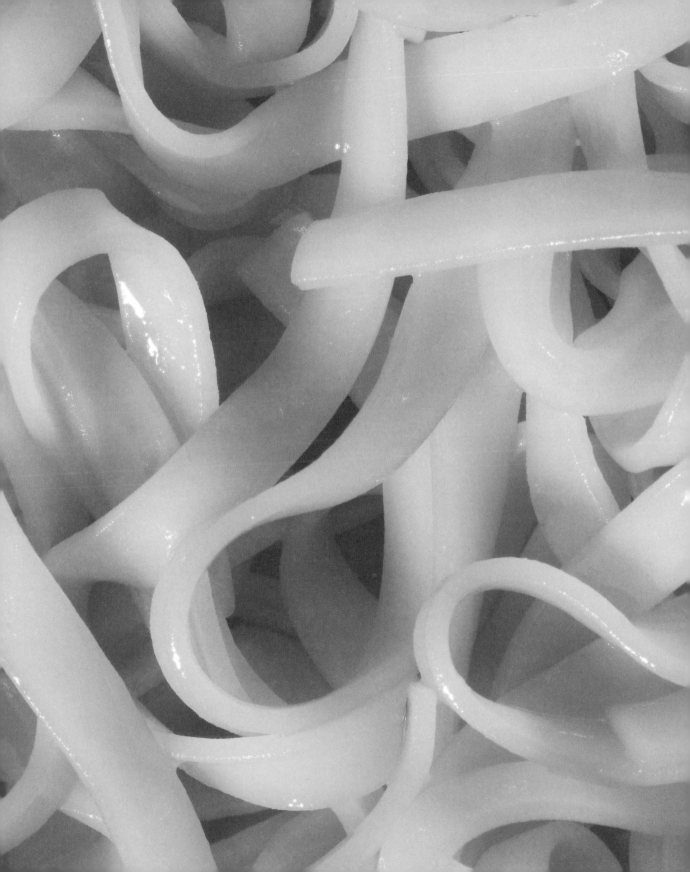

# JAMU NOODLE SOUP

〜〜〜〜〜〜〜〜〜〜〜〜〜〜

## Laksa Paste

100 g (3½ oz) shallots, peeled and roughly chopped

50 g (2 oz) piece of fresh galangal or fresh ginger root, peeled and roughly chopped

50 g (2 oz) piece of fresh turmeric, roughly chopped, or 1 tsp ground turmeric

2 anchovy fillets (tinned in oil)

2 lemongrass stalks, white part only, roughly chopped

2 red bird's eye chillies, roughly chopped (add more to taste)

½ tsp sesame oil

1 tbsp coconut oil

## Noodles

500 g (1 lb 2 oz) dried vermicelli rice noodles

2 handfuls of bean sprouts

## To Serve

soft-boiled eggs (optional)

Balancing Chilli Oil (page 49)

mint leaves

coriander (cilantro)

1 lime, quartered

## Ingredients

### Soup

300 g (10½ oz) raw shell-on prawns (shrimp)

1.5 litres (50 fl oz/6¼ cups) Cure-All Chicken Broth (page 144) or regular chicken stock

400 ml (14 fl oz/1¾ cups) coconut milk

1 tsp sea salt, to taste

1 lemongrass stalk, bashed

1 tbsp tamarind concentrate (or juice of 1 lime)

1 tbsp coconut sugar

Serves 4

**Method**

First prepare the stock for the soup. Peel the prawns (removing the heads too). Keep the prawn meat to one side and fry all the shells and heads in a pot (one that is big enough to accommodate the stock) until they start to take on a wonderful colour and aroma. Pour in the chicken stock and let it simmer gently for 20 minutes or so. If you can't find prawns with their shells on then skip this part.

Put all the laksa paste ingredients, except the coconut oil, in a blender or food processor and blitz to a fine paste.

Melt the coconut oil in a large heavy-based saucepan or stockpot over a high heat, add the laksa paste and fry for 10 minutes until aromatic, then turn off the heat.

Place the noodles and bean sprouts in a heatproof bowl, cover with boiling water and leave to soak for a few minutes until soft. Strain and divide among four bowls.

If you infused your stock with the prawn shells, strain it. Add the stock, coconut milk, salt and bashed lemongrass to the large saucepan or stockpot containing the aromatic laksa paste, turn on the heat to medium and bring to a simmer. Add enough tamarind to the soup to make it pleasantly tangy and simmer for 10 minutes (you may not want to use the whole tablespoon). Add the coconut sugar.

Remove the lemongrass from the soup, add the fresh prawns and simmer for 3–5 minutes until they are cooked through.

Ladle the soup on top of the noodles and bean sprouts, top with the boiled eggs (if using) drizzle with chilli oil and garnish with fresh mint leaves, coriander and lime.

*Recipe photo overleaf*

# TURMERIC AND TAMARIND LAKSA

*This recipe is based on a Nyonya-style laksa, a healing and spicy noodle soup packed with anti-inflammatory ingredients that feature heavily in the traditional system of medicine of Indonesia, known as Jamu (see overleaf).*

JAMU IS A 5,000-YEAR-OLD SYSTEM OF NATURAL HEALING FROM INDONESIA, SIMILAR TO AYURVEDA, THE TRADITIONAL HEALING SYSTEM OF INDIA. IT RELIES SOLELY ON THE POWER OF LOCAL ROOTS, HERBS, SPICES & BARKS TO CURE WHATEVER AILS YOU.

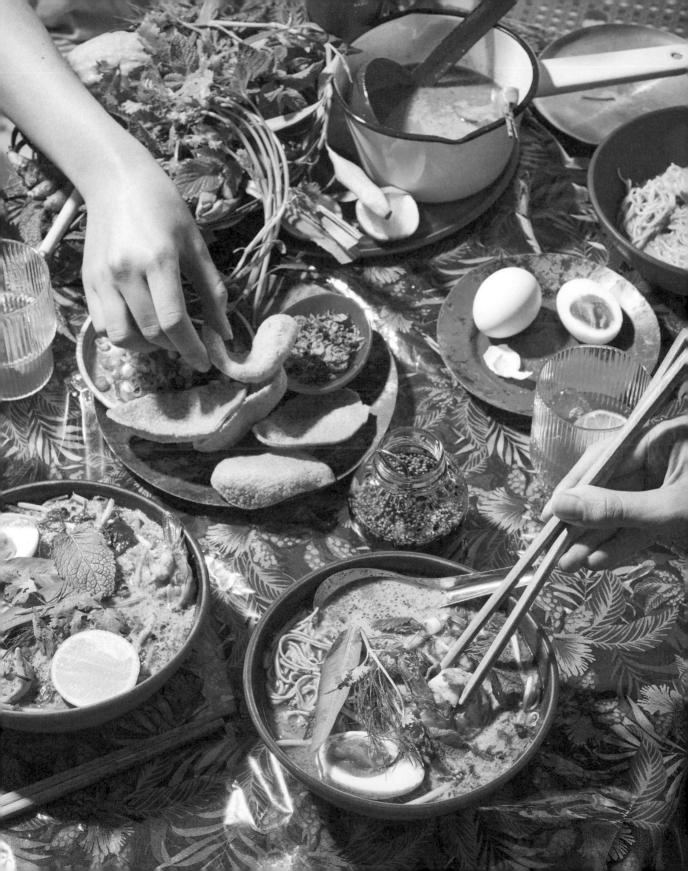

# CURE-ALL CHICKEN BROTH

*If I were to recommend one simple healing food for all-round wellbeing, this **restorative soup tonic** would be it. It's one of the most curative, nutrient-loaded foods a person can consume, and is used by nearly every culture on our planet.*

*According to Chinese medicine, bone broth strengthens and nourishes our kidneys, liver, lungs and spleen, and supports our digestive and immune systems. It's also rich in vitamins, minerals, and collagen, and can be used as a delicious base for soups, congees, stews, sauces, curries or even cooking grains.*

*It's simply made by cooking the bones of healthy animals in water with medicinal roots, vegetables, healing spices, herbs and mushrooms.*

## Method

Put the chicken in a saucepan with enough hot water to cover them, bring to the boil over a high heat, boil for 5 minutes to blanch the meat, then drain and rinse.

Put the blanched chicken and the water in a large saucepan or stockpot and bring to a simmer over a medium heat. Cover and simmer for up to 2 hours, skimming off any foam that appears on the surface.

After 2 hours, turn the heat to low and add the rest of the ingredients. Leave to infuse for at least another hour.

After 3 hours, the broth should have reduced by half. Strain the broth and enjoy it on its own or to use in various other recipes. The broth will keep for 2 days in the fridge. Alternatively, freeze it in portions to use another time.

## Ingredients

750 g (1 lb 10 oz) raw chicken (drumsticks and wings), bashed

3 litres (100 fl oz/12½ cups) water

10 x 10 cm (4 x 4 in) dried kombu sheet

3 tbsp apple cider vinegar

6 dried shiitake mushrooms

2 cm (¾ in) piece of fresh ginger root, smashed

2 cm (¾ in) piece of fresh turmeric, smashed

1 red onion, quartered (with skins)

1 garlic bulb, smashed and peeled

1 red chilli, roughly chopped (with seeds)

1 carrot, chopped

2 spring onions (scallions), washed and chopped

1 celery stick, chopped

1 tbsp whole black peppercorns

**Makes
1.5 litres
(50 fl oz/
6¼ cups)**

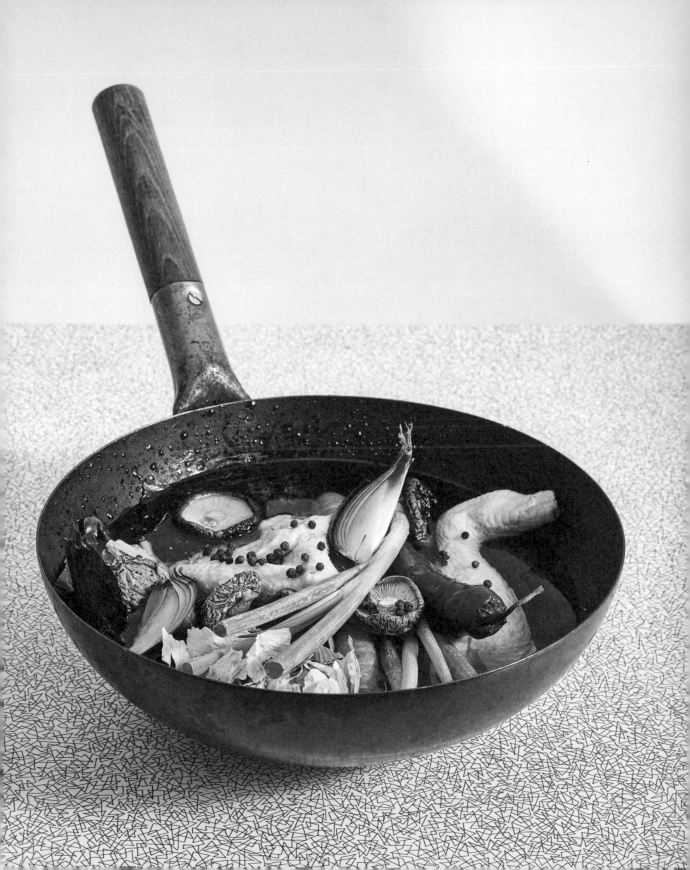

# VEGGIE HEALING BROTH

## BONE-FREE BROTH

*Here's my veggie alternative to the Cure-All Chicken Broth (page 144). It's quicker to make than bone broth, so perfect if you're strapped for time.*

## Method

Pour the water into a large saucepan or stockpot followed by the rest of the ingredients. Stir and bring almost to the boil, then reduce the heat to medium-low and simmer very gently for about 45 minutes.

Strain the broth and enjoy. The broth will keep for 5 days in the fridge. Alternatively, freeze it in portions to use another time.

## Ingredients

3 litres (100 fl oz/12½ cups) water

1 tbsp coconut oil or virgin coconut oil

3 tbsp apple cider vinegar

10 x 10 cm (4 x 4 in) piece of dried kombu sheet

6 dried shiitake mushrooms

2 cm (¾ in) piece of fresh ginger root, smashed

2 cm (¾ in) piece of fresh turmeric, smashed

1 red onion, quartered (with skin)

1 garlic bulb, smashed and peeled

1 red chilli, roughly chopped

1 carrot, chopped

1 leek, washed and chopped

1 celery stick, chopped

1 tbsp whole black peppercorns

**Makes
1.5 litres
(50 fl oz/
6¼ cups)**

**Vegetarian**

**Vegan**

# SUNSHINE CURRY

∿∿∿∿∿∿∿∿∿∿∿

### Ingredients

3 tbsp coconut oil

2 tbsp Invigorating Curry Paste (page 64)

400 ml (14 fl oz) tin of coconut milk

100 ml (3½ fl oz/scant ½ cup) water

½ tbsp fish sauce or lime juice

1 tbsp coconut blossom nectar or any unrefined sugar

300 g (10½ oz) cooked chicken, shredded

2 garlic cloves, sliced

2 tbsp kecap manis (Indonesian sweet soy sauce), or to taste

**Serves 2**

**To make this vegetarian, substitute the chicken with extra veggies and medium-fim tofu, omit the anchovies from the curry paste and sambal and use lime juice**

### To Serve

120 g (4 oz/generous ½ cup) rice of your choice, cooked

handful of spinach

½ cabbage of choice, thinly sliced

1 boiled sweet potato, peeled and cut into chunks

Lemongrass & Ginger Relish (page 60)

Ginger & Tomato Sambal (page 59)

*This anti-inflammatory curry packed with turmeric is inspired by a traditional recipe from Java, Indonesia, known as **opor ayam**. Opor is usually quite soupy, but I prefer a richer, coconutty broth.*

### Method

Melt 1 tablespoon of the coconut oil in a saucepan over a medium heat, add the curry paste and fry for 5 minutes, stirring, until it becomes aromatic. Stir the coconut milk into the paste, little by little, then add the water. Bring to the boil, add the fish sauce or lime juice and sugar to taste, then reduce the heat to low and simmer for about 10 minutes.

Meanwhile, melt the remaining coconut oil in a frying pan (skillet) over a medium heat, add the shredded chicken and garlic and fry until the chicken becomes crispy, then finish with a drizzle of kecap manis.

To serve, layer all of the elements in two bowls. Start with rice, top it with raw spinach and cabbage and sweet potato chunks, then ladle over the curry sauce until it's almost soupy. Top with crunchy chicken. Serve with the lemongrass & ginger relish and ginger & tomato sambal.

*Recipe photo overleaf*

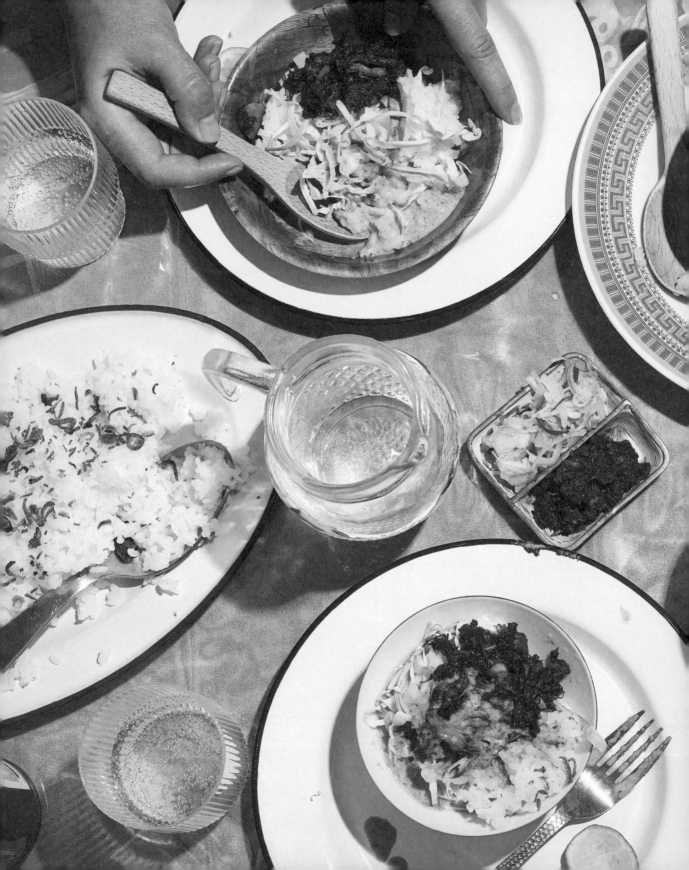

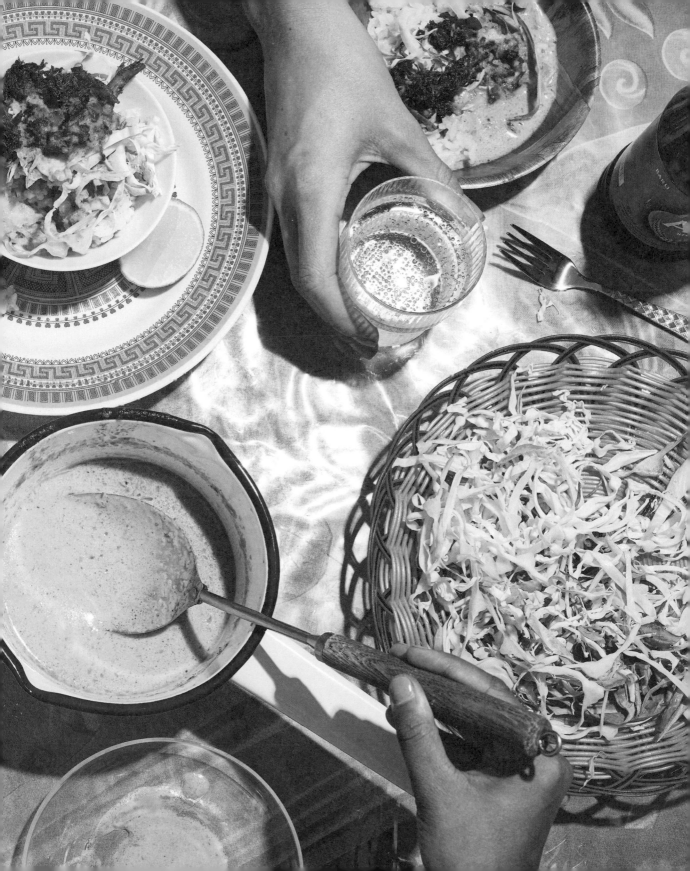

# THE AUTHOR

Author of *Tonic* (Hardie Grant) and chef at London's favourite traditional Japanese udon-ya, Koya Bar, Tanita has an intrepid appetite for all things food and culture, and is on a mission to preserve the traditional values of food cultures that have sustained healthy people for centuries, by linking flavour and fulfilment with health and nature.

Tanita is Dutch by birth, yet her simple approach to health and wellbeing is predominantly inspired by her Mediterranean upbringing in Spain and travels throughout South East Asia as well as Australia.

*'I want to make wellness accessible, and equip people with the education and practical skills they need, without spending much money on products, if any.'*

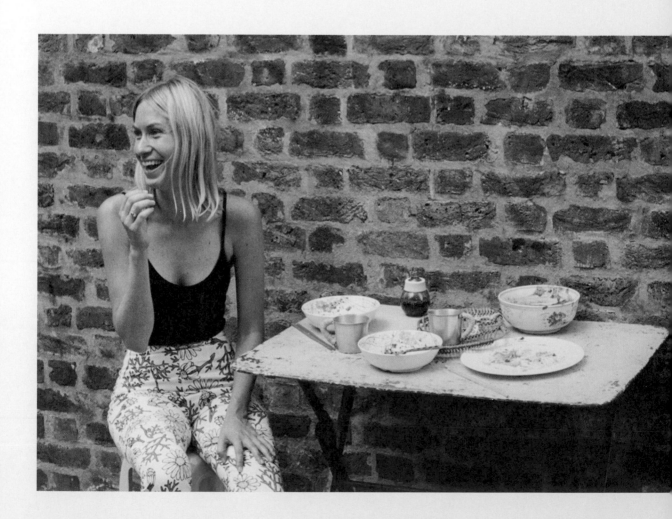

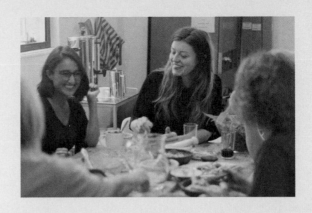

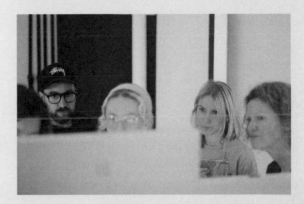

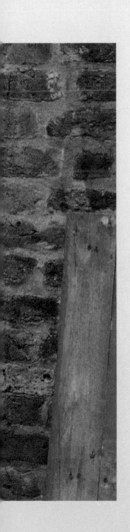

# THANK YOU

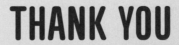

**Forever brilliant & supportive, Dan Buckley** (Design & Direction)
**Most trusting & patient, Kajal Mistry** (Commissioning Editor)
**Loveliest, calmest & cleverest, Patricia Niven** (Photography)
**Most talented & creative, Olivia Bennett** (Stylist)
**Brilliant boyfriend, Gareth Varty** (Always Exciting Film Photography)
**Bestest friend, Tanya Dib** (Chef Assistant)
**Most impressive role model, Eliza Hatch** (Photography Assistant)
**Hardie Grant** (Publisher)

# INDEX

## REFERENCES

**1.** Korean Culture and Information Service (2013) K-food: Combining Flavour, Health, and Nature; Korean Culture, No. 9

**2.** Ho, P. Y. and Lisowki, F. P. (1997) *A Brief History of Chinese Medicine and its Influence*; World Scientific

**3.** Pitchford, P. (2002) *Healing with Whole Foods: Asian Traditions and Modern Nutrition*, North Atlantic Books

**4.** Sho, H. (2001) *History and characteristics of Okinawan longevity food*; Asia Pacific Journal of Clinical Nutrition; Vol. 10, Iss. 2, pp. 159–164

**5.** Soon Hee Kim et al (2016) Korean diet: Characteristics and historical background; *Journal of Ethnic Food*; Vol. 3, Iss. 1, pp. 26–31

Published in 2019 by Hardie Grant Books,
an imprint of Hardie Grant Publishing

Hardie Grant Books (London)
5th & 6th Floors
52–54 Southwark Street
London SE1 1UN

Hardie Grant Books (Melbourne)
Building 1, 658 Church Street
Richmond, Victoria 3121

hardiegrantbooks.com

Copyright text © Tanita de Ruijt
Copyright photography © Patricia Niven

Images on pages 6–7, 14–15 and 150–151
by Gareth Varty

British Library Cataloguing-in-Publication Data.
A catalogue record for this book is available
from the British Library.

Super Roots by Tanita de Ruijt
ISBN: 978-1-78488-241-9

Publishing Director: Kate Pollard
Commissioning Editor: Kajal Mistry
Junior Editor: Eila Purvis
Design & Art Direction: Thumbcrumble.com
Copy Editor: Laura Nickoll
Proofreader: Kay Delves
Photographer: Patricia Niven
Photography Assistant: Eliza Hatch &
Jesse Williams
Retouching: Dark Room Digital
Cover Retoucher: Butterfly Creatives
Food & Prop Stylist: Olivia Bennett
Chef Assistant: Tanya Dib
Indexer: Cathy Heath

Colour Reproduction by p2d
Printed and bound in China by Leo Paper Group